FACELIFTS

FACELIFTS

Everything You Always Wanted to Know

by
Norma Lee Browning

toExcel

San Jose New York Lincoln Shanghai

Facelifts
Everything You Always Wanted to Know

Published by toExcel
an imprint of iUniverse.com, Inc.

For information address:
iUniverse.com, Inc.
620 North 48th Street
Suite 201
Lincoln, NE 68504-3467
www.iuniverse.com

ISBN: 0-595-01054-7

Printed in the United States of America

Contents

PART II

THE FACE PEELERS:
Update

PART III

ROUNDUP TIME
(*Cosmetic Surgery*)

PART IV

LIFT TIPS:
Q & A

PART V

CROSS EXAMINATION:
If You Ask Me, Straight Talk . . .

Acknowledgments

I would like to express my appreciation first of all to the many doctors and patients who contributed so generously of their time and knowledge during the preparation of this book.

Also I had a marvelous team of research assistants. They included Gene Barnes in New York; Susan Nelson and Doris Walsh Erkert in Chicago; Vera Servi and Pam Gallagher in Los Angeles; Caroline Rogers and Maria Rosas in Palm Springs; and Margaret Olwine in Kansas City, Missouri.

I owe a very special debt of gratitude to Mike Kennedy, my former editor on the Chicago *Tribune,* who assigned, encouraged, guided, and trusted me on many forays into fraudulent practices in medicine and other fields.

And a most special thank-you to my editor, Louise Gault, for her patience, perseverance, and guidance in bringing this book to fruition.

Norma Lee Browning

Preface

The Repairman Will Get You
if You Don't Watch Out

With our changing culture and attitudes, cosmetic surgery has come into its own and many people believe that having a facelift will soon become a commonplace beauty procedure, with no more stigma attached to it than having your hair colored or your teeth capped.

Already the booming business in cosmetic surgery has created dissension within the medical profession and a dilemma for those who are giving thoughtful consideration to having a facelift. The biggest risk is not in medical techniques but in the upsurging proliferation of medical interlopers who are not qualified to perform cosmetic surgery.

Today, the public has become very much aware of the importance of getting a *second opinion* before any kind of surgery. It is virtually impossible, however, to get a second opinion with a straight answer in the area of cosmetic surgery.

I hope this book will serve the purpose of a *second opinion* for all of you who may be considering cosmetic surgery of any kind. It is in fact a compilation of many opinions, including my own, after a long arduous tenure of sifting and sorting.

The demand for cosmetic surgery exceeds the supply of qualified cosmetic surgeons, with the result that many patients wind up in the hands of the medical merchandisers with their eyes on the big bucks—and then in the hands of doctors to do the repair work on their botched-up nip-and-tuck jobs.

Many of the doctors and most of the patients I interviewed for this book asked to remain anonymous. I have respected their wishes and used the names only of those who gave permission to do so. This does not imply an endorsement or recommendation of any of the doctors mentioned, although I have chosen to use certain guidelines only from doctors who are widely recognized as authorities in their field.

Given the nature and complexities of cosmetic surgery, it is up to you, the public, to learn to investigate the claims, disregard rhetoric and hype, examine and analyze and choose most cautiously in making the decision that could change your life.

I sincerely hope this book will help you. *Caveat emptor!* And good luck.

> Norma Lee Browning
> Palm Springs, California

FACELIFTS

THE VANITY CRAZE

1

The Great Wrinkle Rip-off

Women are crazy.

They'll do anything to stay young and pretty. Even die for it. Some have. Others almost have.

I've only interviewed the survivors. By and large they're an exuberantly happy breed and ready to swear on a stack of scalpels that the ecstasies far outweigh the agonies, if any, of having a facelift.

One told me cheerfully as she checked in for her lift, "I was going to have it done last year but I had a heart attack on the operating table. So they wouldn't do me."

"Aren't you scared to try it again?" I asked.

She looked at me as if I was the crazy one.

"I've already told them just to go ahead and do me, whatever happens," she said. "So if I drop dead I'll have a new face for my funeral."

True story.

P.S. The lady survived, as most of the facelifted do. The risks are low. Otherwise there wouldn't be about 100,000 people a year flocking to plastic surgeons and face-peelers and forking over $3,000 to $6,000 and up per face—cash in advance, please!—to have their wrinkles removed.

And that's only for your face. When you go in for the bodyworks, the price for resculpting your sags and bags in other areas gets steeper.

But everybody's doing it. Well, almost. A few find other ways of coping with the trauma of growing old. A friend of mine, a handsome young symphony conductor, recently told me, "Turning forty was so traumatic for me that I went out and bought myself a brand-new Porsche."

He could have bought half a dozen facelifts but he figured he didn't need one yet.

Men are more vain than women but they tend to be closet peacocks They're not as open about discussing their facelifts as Betty Ford or Phyllis Diller.

Most women frankly prefer a new face to a new car or a mink coat or a Caribbean cruise, if they can't have them all.

But having a facelift is no longer the special prerogative of the rich and famous. I met one woman who admitted she had mortgaged her farm to pay for her lift.

"I don't plan to grow old gracefully. I'm going to fight it every step of the way," she told me as she sipped vichyssoise through a straw in a fashionable facial rejuvenation salon in Miami. "The smartest thing I ever did was to come here now, when I'm only forty. And when I need it again, I'll come back again. And again and again and again!"

Meanwhile, with her new face she was hoping to find a new husband to pay off her mortgage.

The rejuvenation game has grown into the great All-American Obsession. The facelift has become a status symbol.

As a reporter and longtime observer of the vanity movement in America, I have spent many years investigating and interviewing the lifted and lifters from coast to coast and in other countries as well.

I have personally scrutinized many famous and familiar faces—both before and after their lifts—including those of Phyllis Diller, the zany lady who first brought facelifts out of the closet; Betty Ford, whose much publicized new face launched a new Gold Rush at the overflooded fountains of youth; and Jolie Gabor, who at age 89 has just had her face done again. She had her first lift almost fifty years ago.

Fortunately, I have a ringside seat at one end of this scalpel-happy marathon because I happen to live in Palm Springs, California, which has become the new LIFT capital of the world since Mrs. Ford's facelift caper. People who've been lifted everyplace else, geographically and anatomically, are swarming here like locusts.

But before you cancel your reservation to Rio or Tahiti, keep turning these pages.

You can get a facelift in New York, Chicago, Miami, Memphis, Houston, Dallas, and Des Moines, and most major cities.

There are good and bad doctors in all of them, and in Palm Springs as well.

However, nowhere else have I seen as many before-and-after faces, as many freshly nipped-and-tucked specimens in one spot as in Palm Springs. Many are veteran lift-hoppers, like table-hoppers, blithely doing the cosmetic surgery circuit, going from doctor to doctor in hot pursuit of eternal youth. Some surely would be gold medalists in a facelifting Olympics.

I met one stunning brunette from Kansas City whose lift count—for her face only—must be a record of some sort for her age. She'd just had her *fifth* facelift and she wasn't yet sixty. She'd already had two chemical peels by the top lay operator in Miami and two surgical lifts by nationally known, top-flight plastic surgeons in Kansas City and New York.

She felt she didn't need another peel yet. But she wanted another eye job and some work done on her forehead. She had decided against going back to her doctor in Kansas because "he's too old now." As for the one in New York, "He's too busy to look after his patients. He operated on me one day, then went off to Canada the next day for a meeting."

She had done a lot of "shopping around" for another

plastic surgeon and finally settled for the current new Pygmalion of Palm Springs.

She was recuperating painlessly and ecstatically in the splendiferous surroundings of a hundred-dollar-a-day villa, part of a vast complex reigned over by the Pygmalion, who had just performed her fifth lift.

"He's the greatest," she enthused. "He even tells you how to pluck your eyebrows in a different way so you'll look younger. I'm coming back in a couple of months and have him do my legs. You can't have a doll face with a body falling apart."

Her own doll face could easily have passed for that of a thirty-five- to forty-year-old woman. So could her body as far as I could tell, and she was bent on keeping it that way.

"I love swimming and tennis and I'm getting a little flabbiness on my inner thighs. I want it off before it becomes too noticeable. There'll be scars but they'll be inside and eventually they will go away," she said.

Her doctor was one who specializes in all-over bodyworks as well as faces. He is frequently the guest of honor at "unveiling" parties hosted by his happy clients to show off their new faces.

Unveiling parties are quite common in Palm Springs and plastic surgeons are very much a part of the social scene.

I've been to more unveiling parties than I can count. It's amazing how eager people are to show off their various face and body jobs and the lifters who did them.

"Look at my eyes. Aren't they gorgeous! *He* did them," says the hostess, while He beams and lines up more clients.

At one party a forty-year-old woman came up to me and bubbled, "He's done me all over, my eyes, my nose, my chin. But not only my face. I mean everything. My boobs, belly, thighs, fanny, the whole works."

She insisted on showing me. I told her I'd take a rain check on it.

At another unveiling a young man approached me and

said, rather abruptly, I thought, "Take a good look at my nose."

Well . . .

"He did it," he said, nodding toward the guest of honor. "You know why I like his noses? Because they don't look like a Dr. X nose." (He used the doctor's name.)

In chic lifting circles, it is commonplace to hear remarks that can be taken as either catty or complimentary, depending on your point of view, such as, "Oh, you can tell it's a So-and-so nose." Or a Smith chin. Or a Jones eye job. It's like recognizing a Chanel suit when you see one.

Some doctors turn out noses, chins, or eye jobs that all look the same. The "in" people can tell immediately who did them. Some clients don't mind this, particularly if the doctor happens to be famous for noses. (Or eyes, etcetera.) Others, like the young man talking to me, have a different point of view. *"He* does noses to fit your face. My nose looks like me," he said proudly. I was willing to take his word for it since I had never met him before. He introduced himself. He was an attorney, forty-three years old. He said he didn't like his old nose so he just decided to have a new one.

He gave me his card, adding that he'd be delighted to give me a written testimonial for his doctor. I took a rain check on that too.

At the same party, four newly remodeled women, all from out of state, stampeded me with raving testimonials for the plastic surgeon who had performed their assorted body jobs.

I have heard equally raving hosannas for everyone from Dr. A to Z, clear through the alphabet and back again.

But if Dr. X is the "in" facelifter this season, he could very well be "out" by next season.

Much depends on WHO is going to WHOM. It's a form of Russian roulette called Follow the Leader.

Only a few seasons ago, for example, I went to an unveiling luncheon party for one of Jolie Gabor's facelifts. That one was done by Dr. X, who was considered *the* best "Face Man" in Palm Springs at the time and Mr. Kingpin of the Carriage

Trade. Now he's "out" and the new Dr. X kingpin is "in," so Jolie had her most recent lifts done by him—though by the time this is in print, he may be *out* and a new one *in*. The same as in fashions or hairstyles, facelifting is trendy as far as facelifters go.

Though most people credit Phyllis Diller and Betty Ford for bringing facelifts out of the closet by going public with them, Jolie Gabor claims she was the real pioneer by having her first facelift when she was only forty years old. (More or less.)

"Dahlink, you know *I* vas ze pioneer of thees facelift business," she told me recently. "He vas ze most famous doc-toor in New York who give me ze first facelift."

He was indeed the most famous "face man" of the time, long before the vanity craze came out in the open.

All of the Gabors, of course, are totally dedicated to staying young and beautiful. Their total lift count is probably exceeded only by their collective total of husbands and lovers. But Jolie's marriages last longer than those of her daughters. Her last unveiling party was a very glamorous affair also celebrating her twenty-third wedding anniversary. (She is married to a former Hungarian Count, Edmond DeSzigethy.)

Jolie once traded a Polish count for a rhinestone bathing suit. Her goals and lifestyle haven't changed much. The first time I met her, she told me I should be a blonde and wear false eyelashes. She gave me one of Eva's wigs and a couple of boxes of eyelashes. They didn't do much for me so I gave up on them. Later, she gave me another wig, more eyelashes, and said, "So, dahlink, now tell me, vy do you not have also thees facelift?"

A good question. I'll come to that later.

Jolie has no intention of growing old. If she has to die she hopes only that it won't happen while she's taking a bath and not wearing her false eyelashes. Each time she steps in the tub she says a little prayer, "Please, God, do not let me die in ze tub without my eyelashes."

She still jogs and swims daily, goes bowling, dancing, and

partying with great fervor, speaks deliciously of Sex After Sixty, and is always the life of the party in her low-cut gowns, ostrich feathers, false eyelashes, and new face. She's the sexiest, youngest-at-heart, and most glamorous of all the Gabors.

At nearly ninety we should all look as good as Jolie!

Not everyone is as totally dedicated to staying young and beautiful as the Gabors.

But most women, if they're completely honest about it, are in the same vanity boat when they look in the mirror. How often have you wished that those wrinkles would just zap off and fly away?

So okay, call them "character lines" if you wish.

Some might call that wishful thinking or self-delusion.

And many take big risks to try to turn back the age clock. In Chicago I met a pretty, freshly peeled jet-setter, one of JFK's former girl friends, who recounted her harrowing experience with two quacks in a face-peel factory in Connecticut.

"The pain was unbearable and I got so scared I wouldn't let them do my neck. But now I wish I had," she told me. She knew the peel parlor had been closed, the operation was dangerous, but still she said, "So I'm alive and beautiful, I don't have any scars, I look at least ten years younger. I know it's crazy but I'd be willing to take the same risk again. That's how vain we are."

Not all vain people are flea brains. A female college professor in her early forties put it this way, "I wanted my eyes fixed and my face lifted because I'm vain and I want to look young for as long as I can. Is that so terrible?"

My friend Rose Wilder Lane, the novelist, a brilliant intellectual heavyweight, decided at age seventy-four that she wanted to have her face lifted—and also her hands and arms even more.

She wrote to a Miami rejuvenator: "If I must, I can be reconciled to a drooping face because, as some versifier put it, 'My face I don't mind it because I'm behind it; it's the people

in front that I jar.' But I see my hands, I can hardly avoid seeing them most of the time prancing over the typewriter keys,
and they make me sick. I mean damn annoyed."

The operator didn't want to take a chance on a woman of
Mrs. Lane's age and temperament, tried to discourage her with
high fees, warnings of pain and discomfort, the necessity of a
complete physical examination.

Mrs. Lane balked at this. "In general I do not like nor
trust doctors," she said. She hadn't consulted a doctor since
1921 when she was in Constantinople and American doctors
there had prescribed sixty grains of quinine daily for her ma-
laria, which made her unconscious by noon every day. She
insisted on having her face, arms, and hands done.

"I am not too badly wrinkled but neck- and jawlines are
becoming turkey-gobblerish and my upper eyelids sag. The
eyelids are annoying, slightly uncomfortable, and I would
enjoy a smooth neck, a clear jawline, and firmer cheeks again
as well as hands that are not so unbearable."

In the end they compromised. Mrs. Lane, an inveterate
rebel, grudgingly submitted to a physical by a bona fide MD to
have her face, hands, and arms peeled by lay operators with a
chemical-acid process that was then being blasted by the medical profession.

It's all the vogue now and the MDs who hard-sell patients
on a peel as an "adjunct" to plastic surgery facelifts are using
the same formula with a little bit more or less of this and that
which they once said would kill you, or at least burn your face
off.

Trends change. Today the Peel is Trendy. (See Chapters
8–11.)

Despite dire predictions, Rose Wilder Lane survived
splendidly for twelve years—to age eighty-six—immensely enjoying her smooth neck, clear jawline, firmer cheeks, de-
wrinkled arms and hands prancing over her typewriter. The
last time I saw her (1972), she was in glowing health and
packing up her bags and typewriter for another extended so-

journ abroad. Her only complaint against her de-wrinkling treatment was that it required a pre-peel examination by an MD!

My odyssey through the Fountain-of-Youth Fantasyland has led me to one certain conviction which is the reason for this book:

The vanity craze has created utter confusion among the masses and such cutthroat competition among the scalpel wielders that it leaves a lot of us asking—

SHOULD I or *SHOULDN'T I?????*

Apart from the crazies who will pay any price, undergo any pain, take any risk to turn the clock back, there are still many of us more or less so-called average or normal people who would simply like to know whether it's worth it to have a facelift.

This book is for you.

Facelifts will soon be as commonplace as changing your hair or having your teeth capped. The clientele of the youth doctors is becoming increasingly comprised of non-celebrities —housewives, secretaries, bank clerks, airline hostesses, pilots, gas station attendants, policemen, and truck drivers. The growing acceptance of plastic surgery by the average man and woman means they're no longer waiting to be sold on the idea; they've already been sold. Now they want answers to specific questions.

In the jungleland of questions and answers, it's a world strewn with wall-to-wall contradictions from wall-to-wall rip-off artists cashing in on the youth boom.

Don't panic. By this I do not mean they're out to rip off any part of your anatomy and leave you physically impaired or mutilated. This rarely happens, although it can. Remember the case of the misplaced belly button which caused a New York plastic surgeon some problems? He allegedly misplaced the lady's navel by two inches during a tummy-tightening operation and a jury awarded her $854,219 for the mishap. The wandering omphalos was put back in place by a repairman (repair jobs are booming) with an explanation from the aggrieved forty-two-year-old claimant: "A centered belly button is a valuable feminine attribute. Singer Cher made millions on hers."

A facelift entails fewer risks. But it is by no means risk-free. (For specifics see Chapters 12 and 20.)

Some experts will tell you there is no more risk in having your face lifted than there is when you're flying or having a root canal job in your dentist's chair. Others say it's as risky as any type of major surgery. Which of the experts are we to believe?

Some say it's dangerous to have your lower eyelids done, others say it isn't. Some claim it's better to do the eyes, nose, and face separately; others insist on doing the whole surgical enchilada at the same time. Some operate only in a hospital, others only in their offices. Many cosmetic surgeons perform chemical peels along with surgery; others recommend the peel a month or two after surgery; still others won't do it at all.

The most honest plastic surgeon of the many I've interviewed was the one who, when I asked why he didn't do peels, replied, "Because I'm not qualified."

The medical literature is filled with pompous pronouncements on the vital importance of your *MOTIVATION* for a facelift. Do you want it because you're trying to hold a husband or a lover? Or find one? Or for other allegedly "neurotic" reasons? Tsk, tsk, say the experts, many of whom fancy themselves as mind doctors.

I have posed as a facelift candidate for scores of doctors. None has ever asked, *"Why* do you want a facelift?" It's usually *when?* If I back out, it's usually, "Why don't you want it?"

Obviously I need it, as many of the top drawer lifters have told me. Many of them I wouldn't let touch my face with a ten-foot pole.

You'd be surprised how many free facelifts I've been offered by doctors I've interviewed for this book.

When I've found the right doctor, I'll pay my own way,

thanks. And this is the crux of the dilemma for most of us. Finding the right doctor is going to require a lot of soul-searching as well as sole-treading.

Most of the experts start off by telling you to ask your "family physician" and/or your local medical society.

So what if your family physician is a squarehead who doesn't believe in facelifts? And your local medical society gives you the usual run-around with the names of three doctors who turn out to be specialists in another field?

Unfortunately, in most states any MD can, quite legally, set up shop as a plastic surgeon. Many are doing just that. The field is inundated with surgeons of all stripes who have discovered that cosmetic surgery is more lucrative than their original specialty. Many ear, nose, and throat (ENT) specialists now call themselves "face and neck" doctors and do everything in the plastic surgery field in that area—noses, facelifts, hair transplants, etcetera.

Urologists, dermatologists, and neurologists have hopped on the body-beautiful bandwagon. Betty Ford's gynecologist reportedly assisted with her facelift. It was widely circulated that she had to have a repair job on her face.

All the alleged repairmen of course hotly denied doing it.

As one of them told me, "I wouldn't touch her face for a million dollars—not with all of her personal problems."

He added bluntly, "And furthermore I'm sick of all this prostitution of plastic surgery. I'm thinking seriously of getting out of the business." (In my opinion he should!) "Everyone is getting into the act and they don't know anything about faces. Would you trust your face to a man who specializes in gall bladders? The trouble is, they've all got dollar signs in their eyes. It's a rip-off."

I've heard the same complaint from practically every facelifter I've talked to.

Paradoxically, complaints from patients are rare; they don't seem to mind being ripped off in the pocketbook as long as they come out looking good.

Therefore, plastic surgery is probably the most competitively cutthroat branch of medicine and the plastic surgeons reserve their most dedicated wielding of the knife for each other.

In brief, they are generally the most jealous, narcissistic, and egomaniacal bunch of prima donnas in the business. Some even admit it. I know a lot of them won't take kindly to these words.

But I'm not writing this book for the doctors. I'm writing it for those people who are trying to make up their minds whether to have a facelift. I happen to be one of them. As far as I'm concerned, the biggest risk is the rip-off. I certainly wouldn't want my wrinkles removed by a doctor who does gall bladders. Would you?

2

"I'll Give You a Nose Just Like Betty Ford's"

(The Truth Behind Betty's Facelift Caper)

I'm sure no one was surprised when Betty Ford, who has never been one to shy away from making public statements on her personal problems, happily announced in September of 1978 why she'd had a facelift:

"I'm sixty years old and I wanted a new face to go with my beautiful new life."

Those famous words and her famous new face made front-page headlines everywhere, and while you may or may not think her facelift is so ginger peachy, you can take a few tips from the behind-the-scenes controversy it left in its wake.

From all the furor it created, you'd think Betty Ford invented the facelift. She didn't. Nor was her "unveiling" the first one in Palm Springs. They've been going on here for years.

Mrs. Ford's unveiling, however, was the most auspicious and the most expensive one I've ever attended.

Officially it was a fund-raising event for the desert's Theater of Performing Arts and presented as a "Musical Salute to Betty Ford . . . for her interest in the arts and her contribution toward human understanding." (She's the theater's patron chairman.)

But it was her first post-lift public appearance and the thousand or so gaping guests were far less concerned with theater and the arts than with Betty's new face.

Moreover, they paid plenty to get a good squint at it.

A privileged few coughed up $1,000 each to sit at the same luncheon table with Mrs. Ford.

Those with $25 "Silver" tickets got only a long-shot view of her during the drawn-out program in the Grand Ballroom of Marriott's Rancho Las Palmas Resort in Rancho Mirage.

The $100 "Gold" ticket holders got the close-up view at a private fruit-punch reception preceding the luncheon. The former First Lady stood for an hour shaking hands, chitchatting, graciously posing for photographers, and gallantly exposing her new face to the scrutiny of a mob of nit-picky females absorbed in ferreting out the flaws and comparing her nose and eye job and jowl line with their own and everybody else's in the room.

Luckily, I had latched on to a "Gold" ticket, which got me a ringside seat next to her luncheon table as well as an eyeball-to-eyeball chat with her at the reception.

Jolie Gabor almost stole the show from Betty. She made her own grand entrance, wearing boots, cape, a cocky-floppy big beret, and sharing her dashing escort, Beau James, with Elizabeth Taylor's beautiful mother, Sara.

Naturally, the nit-pickers had a ball comparing Jolie's face with Mrs. Ford's. "Watch their eyes when they smile. That's how you tell. Jolie doesn't have as many wrinkles as Betty." Tsk, tsk.

The fund-raiser raised a lot of money for the theater and a lot of eyebrows over Betty Ford's new total image.

Some thought she looked fabulous, others thought her facelift was dreadful.

The vote was split on whether it was her new face or her new hair-do and makeup that had changed her image. Most agreed that her new short-cropped, upswept casual hairstyle was far more becoming than the old bouffant she used to wear, which gave her a hydrocephalic look.

Inevitably it stirred up a great debate over who did the most for Betty Ford's new face—her facelifter or her hairdresser.

She didn't ask me, but personally I'd opt for her hairdresser and her professional makeup job.

Having seen Mrs. Ford at various functions, and occasionally chatting with her briefly, I was certainly aware of the spectacular change in her total look after her facelift.

But it was not the facelift alone that changed her.

This is the important point for all of you who are considering a facelift to remember—

Do not expect your facelifter to perform miracles.

A great deal depends on your hairstyle, your makeup, your weight, your dress, your carriage, and your mental attitude.

Actually, Mrs. Ford's so-called fabulous facelift was only a small part of a complete psychological recycling to create a new image to go with her "beautiful new life," as she herself put it.

Of course public figures such as Mrs. Ford are always in the limelight and subject to closer scrutiny than the average Mrs. John Doe. Inevitably, the rumors began flying as thick as desert jack rabbits. *Her chin is slipping. Her face is too tight. Her right eye is drooping. Her nose bob is for the birds. Her wrinkles are back.*

It became an open secret that Mrs. Ford had gone to another doctor for a repair job.

It was also an open secret that something had gone wrong during her facelift operation and another doctor was called in to assist in the operation. The assistant reportedly was her gynecologist.

These reports were never confirmed nor denied.

Meanwhile, phones were ringing off the hooks in Palm Springs with calls from facelift candidates all over the world wanting Betty Ford's doctor. But they couldn't get him. He was booked up six months in advance, had increased his fees, and besides, he said, he didn't want their business anyway.

There were other doctors just as good or better than he was, he modestly proclaimed, and if he had known what he was getting into with Mrs. Ford, he wouldn't have done her.

The $64 question was why he did; and why she picked him over other qualified cosmetic surgeons.

Mrs. Ford had consulted other doctors about a facelift before she went into the Long Beach Naval Hospital for her drug and alcohol addiction problem in April 1978.

They refused to take her at that time because, as one of them told me, "It was not the right time. I wouldn't do a facelift on any woman with the personal problems and emotional stress and strain that Mrs. Ford was going through at the time."

Charges, counter-charges, and questions peppered the scenario: Why did she spend a week in Eisenhower Hospital for a five-and-a-half-hour facelift that normally requires only three and a half hours and an overnight stay? Why did she choose an unknown Iranian who had never operated at Eisenhower before? (And hasn't since.)

The consensus among other facelifters was that he was the only one who would take her—or who had the time open for her cosmetic surgery when she wanted it.

Most of the plastic surgeons I talked to agreed that the period immediately before or after a drug and alcohol therapy program such as Mrs. Ford went through—and not of her own volition but under duress—is the *wrong* time to have a facelift.

It's easy to picture the emotional wringing she was going through in the hospital. She no doubt made her facelift decision impulsively, saying to herself, By golly, now is the time, I am going to have it done!

We have all made such rash and hasty decisions.

Obviously, Mrs. Ford made up her mind she was going to have a facelift—and like a lot of women, whether it was the right time or wrong time—and she found a doctor who would do it in spite of her personal problems.

It's an open secret that she made her decision based upon the recommendation of her hairdresser and gynecologist. (Personally, I'd say your hairdresser knows more about your face than your gynecologist.)

Several doctors were involved in the hush-hush imbroglio. One of them told me, "It's a rip-off, one of the biggest cons in medical history."

He was referring specifically to the before-and-after pictures of Betty Ford, widely circulated in newspapers and magazines, which deluded thousands of women into thinking it was her facelift that made the difference.

Bona fide Betty-watchers knew better. Most of them would tell you they never saw her look *that* bad before nor *that* good after—as the before-and-after photographs portrayed her.

The popular platitude that photographs don't lie is a myth. Everyone knows that photographs *can* lie and often do, by shading the truth with proper lighting and makeup, by retouching, by catching a subject at certain flattering or unflattering angles. The camera lens can pick up and magnify or distort details which the human eye does not see.

Before-and-after *facelift* photographs are especially notorious for accentuating the negative and embellishing the positive. Getting before-and-after pictures is part of the routine procedure for many plastic surgeons, often for their own medical files and technical papers—or to impress prospective clients.

I have seen literally thousands of before-and-after facelift pictures showing transformations as seemingly miraculous as Mrs. Ford's—including one who turned out to be a good friend of mine. The doctor projected her before-and-after blow-ups on his big clinic screen; I didn't recognize her in *either* picture, even after he told me who she was.

I have also seen many "before" pictures of Mrs. Ford that were just as flattering as those with her "new face"—including some taken at another theater luncheon which I attended a few months before she had her facelift. I sat directly across the table from her during a press interview. Her "before" face looked fine then. The consensus among those who know her best and have seen her the most is that Betty Ford didn't need a facelift; she had it to uplift her spirits and morale when she was going through an emotional crisis—and it apparently worked wonders for her in spite of the fact that some doctors said it was the "wrong" time for her to have a facelift.

There is no question that Mrs. Ford looks younger, prettier, more vivacious, and happier today than she did ten years ago, as millions know who have seen her on television.

She looks great, she looks spectacular—are comments frequently heard wherever she goes.

Unfortunately, many attribute the drastic change in her looks only to her highly publicized facelift.

They forget that there were many other factors involved in her total new look.

Doctors were suddenly besieged by women who had seen Betty Ford's before-and-after facelift photographs—and who were deluded into thinking they could achieve a similarly drastic and dramatic change in their looks by merely having a facelift.

Typical were some of the facelift candidates I met when I went to see Mrs. Ford's doctor. It took me two months to get an appointment for a consultation with him, and then another two hours of waiting for him to show up at his office.

By then I already knew we weren't meant for each other. In fact, I knew it the minute I stepped inside his cubbyhole waiting room.

His operations are routinely performed in the back rooms of his office, or "clinic," though Mrs. Ford's was performed in a hospital. I'm sure she never set foot in his office, or she would have waltzed right out again.

The waiting room was jammed with eager ladies-in-waiting to be lifted. There was a steady traffic jam at two open-window counters where a couple of white-frocked aides took the money-down deposits, scheduled the dates for surgery, and dispersed instructions of a very private and confidential nature within earshot of all of us.

Each woman was given a pre-operative briefing on her medication, vitamins, laxatives, Betadine shampoo, Phisohex and anti-bacterial soap, as well as her Cryogel ice bags and Mary Jane bra.

You could tell from the dialogue which ones were candidates for facelifts, breast surgery, chin or cheek augmentation.

On one side of me sat an attractive blond woman who told me she had driven over from San Diego especially for her consultation.

"Why did you come here when you have good plastic surgeons in San Diego?" I asked.

She appeared genuinely startled at the question.

"Well! I think this man did a fantastic job on Mrs. Ford's face, don't you?"

On the other side of me was a rather frumpy, middle-aged woman from Idaho who had just landed in Palm Springs and had come straight from the airport to the doctor's office, she said, because this was Saturday, the doctor's only consultation day during the week, and he had already scheduled her surgery for Monday morning.

Most plastic surgeons claim to have at least one, usually more, consultations with clients before accepting (or rejecting) them for cosmetic surgery.

The truth is that some practically hog-tie you to a money-down contract without a first or second look at your face.

The woman from Idaho was having her very first consultation with the doctor on Saturday afternoon, with her operation already scheduled for Monday morning.

I couldn't believe that anyone would have a facelift—or any kind of operation, for that matter—from a doctor she had never met.

When I expressed my amazement, she glowered at me as though I belonged in the loony bin, and said huffily, "Well! If he's good enough for Betty Ford, he's good enough for me."

When my name was called, I followed the doctor into a small office dominated by a big cluttered desk and an assortment of sketch pads. He spent 90 per cent of our consultation time telling me how terrible all the other plastic surgeons were and how great he was; the other 10 per cent of the time he made quickie pencil sketches of my face, section by section, on his sketch pads, and marked down a price tag for each section.

He told me what was wrong here and there, what I needed, and what he could do for me. He finally worked up to the denouement:

"I'll give you a tipped nose just like Betty Ford's."

I was a bit jolted. My nose isn't the greatest but I've never given it much thought. Other wrinkle removers have volunteered all sorts of advice about my face but none before or since has tried to sell me on a nose job too.

I was further intrigued by the dizzying speed with which the doctor added up the cost figures. They came to $4,800.

"That's with the 20 per cent discount," he said.

"What's the discount for?"

"That's if you have it all done in one operation. The regular fee is $6,000 if I do the face and nose separately," he explained.

At the check-out counter where I paid my $35 consultation fee, the aide thumbed through her appointment book and said brightly, "Well, aren't you lucky. The doctor just happens to have an opening. . . . Would you like to schedule your surgery now?"

A $300 deposit was required within two weeks.

I politely demurred. Even at a 20 per cent discount I didn't want a nose just like Betty Ford's. And this is not to disparage her nose. I think it's a lovely nose.

But I'm allergic to fast-sell jobs, whether it's noses or magazine subscriptions.

For all of you who are considering a facelift—or any other kind of lift—here are some important lift tips to remember:

• Do *not* count on your doctor to do a quickie make-over and remodel you to look like Betty Ford, Elizabeth Taylor, the

Gabors, or Sophia Loren. It can't be done. You start with what you have. No way can the woman from Idaho, for instance, get the spectacular results she expects without a lot of shaping up in other directions.

• Do *not* base your decision for a facelift on before-and-after pictures. (For more details on this see Chapter 14.)

• Do *not* be influenced by celebrity status seekers—the lifters who like to boast about the famous movie stars they've done. (As well as political and sports celebrities.)

• Do *not* have a facelift just because all the VIPs are doing it; make sure it's because *you* want it.

And for heaven's sake, don't get yourself locked in with a lifter who guarantees you a nose just like Bob Hope's.

3

Palm Springs:

The New Mecca for Facelifts

Are Palm Springs doctors any better?

I can't vouch for that but they certainly are more esoteric and avant-garde.

There are some heady fringe benefits that come with a Palm Springs facelift.

The opulent desert oasis of course is known as one of the world's choicest playgrounds of the rich and famous. It's a gold-plated watering hole with an elegantly nutty and laid-back lifestyle, a microcosm of all those things you've always heard about Hollywood and Southern California where, according to widespread reports, approximately 97.8 per cent of the inhabitants are irreversibly crazy.

It's a result of the Life-Is-a-Lark syndrome and is commonly called Doing Your Own Thing.

So naturally, no one expects doctors in Palm Springs to follow the AMA's manual for decorum as they do in more conservative cities.

It's the only place I've ever been, for instance, where MDs practice medicine by telephone from their Rolls-Royce golf carts, and facelifters treat you to a slice of the Good Life after sloping off your sags and bags—in a beautiful and glamorous setting that looks like a Hollywood backdrop with lots of exotic trappings.

Most of our facelifters are very social. They may invite you to luncheon or cocktails in their home. They may even have an unveiling party for you (or let you have one for them).

You'll never need to feel embarrassed or stay in the closet with your newly lifted or peeled face, even if it's still black and blue. It's the most out-in-the-open topic of conversation. You'll find the shopkeepers very helpful with advice—or inquisitive about how you liked Dr. So-and-so. Most of them have already had facelifts, the others are in the market for one, and all of them are quite accustomed to the everyday passing parade of lifted ladies in their Oscar de la Renta head scarves and sunglasses that are merely part of the Palm Springs scenery, as commonplace as the jack rabbits that dot the desert landscape and the multimillionaires who tool around bumper to bumper in their Rolls-Royce golf carts.

In Palm Springs a facelift is as taken-for-granted as a Gucci tote bag.

This may be the main reason it has become the new mecca for facelifts—and for facelifters cashing in on the cosmetic surgery boom.

Generally, the medical background of a facelifter in Palm Springs has very little, if anything, to do with a person's choice of that doctor.

Some are not qualified plastic surgeons. Some are not qualified. Period.

Still, people flock here not only for their facelifts, but for the climate, the scenery, the people-watching, and the sybaritic Good Life that goes along with the lift. (If you can afford it.)

First of all, you will not need to check into a hospital. In Palm Springs, facelifters shun hospitals like poison. They operate in their own offices, now called "private clinics." This trend is much more prevalent on the West Coast than in the East.

As one lifter told me, "I don't believe in doing facelifts in hospitals. If a patient gets stuck in a room with someone who's had a hysterectomy or a rectal operation, she could get a staph infection just from the environment. It can't be sterile. It's much safer to do a facelift in this kind of setting." (His office.)

Another important consideration is—what type of post-surgery recovery facilities are provided for patients who've had facelifts?

In Palm Springs you go to a plush resort hotel, a $100-a-day condominium, a villa, or an exotic "recovery ranch," depending on whether you've been lifted by Dr. W, X, Y, or Z.

One doctor treats his lifted patients to the Good Life on his recovery ranch near Rancho Mirage, which features informal boudoirs clustered around his skinny-dipping pool, an arabesque sauna house, an organic garden, and a lot of strange livestock, mostly llamas and camels, ranging around beside an artificial duck pond.

"I'd rather have a camel than a Rolls-Royce," the lifter says seriously. "They don't eat all that much and they're nice to have around as conversation pieces."

Inside his sheikish desert homestead, freshly lifted patients waiting for their stitches to come out lounge around on Turkish floor pillows, surrounded by primitive wooden icons from New Guinea (the doctor travels a lot), reading *The Sensuous Woman,* or meditating. The post-op regimen includes meditation periods and an organic diet for beautification of the body. The lifter does an occasional nose job and fanny augmentation, but his biggest trade is in rejuvenating sagging breasts and faces, many of them for Las Vegas showgirls.

Whatever appendage his hands have molded back into shape, the appendage owners are usually pleased.

He permits his patients to start swimming the third day after surgery. On any day during the winter resort season, you can see torsos sautéeing in cocoa butter around his recovery-ranch pool. On the day I visited, one woman, naked and pan-fried from stem to stern except for gobs of masking tape around her convalescing breasts, exclaimed rapturously, "It's heaven! So what the hell—if I get wrinkles, I'll come back and let him do my face."

Practically all doctors everywhere agree too much sun is bad for you—except those who practice in Palm Springs where the sun shines most of the time.

As one told me, "This is the best place in the world to practice plastic surgery because Mother Nature is on my side. Patients heal about one third faster here. The air is sterile, the climate dry. . . . It's the sun and air and dry climate that make healing faster."

This particular doctor advises his patients to wait two weeks before going swimming, golfing, horseback riding, etcetera, but most of them don't pay any attention to him.

A friend of mine stopped by to show me her new face, only a week old. She was in her tennis clothes and on her way to the Racquet Club for a breakfast and tennis date with her boyfriend. After that, they were going horseback riding.

The lifestyle of Palm Springs lifters blends in well with the flamboyant kitsch of the super-rich. Most of them have become super-rich themselves in a very short time. They're plucking up property as madly as the Saudis in Beverly Hills. Some of their homes are not to be believed. One has a multimillion-dollar bachelor pad, complete with indoor waterfall and lily pond, just a couple of pinyon clumps down from Bob Hope's mountaintop Taj Mahal. It's famous for its social soirées and unveiling parties where the doctor exhibits his newly lifted specimens.

His A-1 competitor does his own thing in a rather far-out bubble-top house where clients are wooed with homemade Persian goodies and catered shish kebab. And *their* A-1 competition does his thing on a seven-acre ranch with goats and horses. When you go to his "clinic" for a consultation, you're greeted by a guy in white surgical cap and gown, blue jeans, and fresh-from-the-ranch cowboy boots.

Another doctor's working wardrobe runs to colorful tunics

from the South Seas and Bali. He's listed in the Social Register and has as big a reputation as a socialite as a surgeon.

He hires a top society photographer to shoot his more dramatic operations and a publicist to get his name in print.

His colleagues call him a "publicity seeker," which is like the pot calling the kettle black.

Most Palm Springs facelifters are adept at the art of hustling. One even grabbed me by the coattail at a recent soirée and asked when I was coming in to see him.

There are several current darlings on the desert's facelift circuit, all vying for the title of King of Plastic Surgery for the Beautiful People set, and loosely bandying about the names of celebrities they've lifted.

I asked a friend of mine why she chose a certain facelifter and she said, "I heard he did Frank Sinatra's face. If he's good enough for Sinatra, he's good enough for me." (No one has confirmed whether Sinatra has had a facelift.)

Did she like her face? "No. He didn't take enough off. But he's going to do it over."

About 99.9 per cent of the lifted ladies in Palm Springs are 100-per-cent-satisfied customers but about 99.9 per cent of the ones I've met also make at least one or two return trips to the lifter's office for a little repairwork here or there.

Most of the 100-per-cent-satisfied customers don't seem to mind the inadequate care and service they often get in their $100- or $150-per-day recovery facilities. It takes a lot to disenchant a lady with a lifter who can put a twenty-five-year-old face on her seventy-year-old body.

I know one woman who paid $6,000 for her transformation, then $150 a day to recuperate in her lifter's villa. It had a marvelous mountain view but no bath towels for a week. Did it bother her? Not at all. "I had three washcloths," she told me. And she loves her face. That's what counts.

I visited one freshly lifted and peeled client in her $100-a-day doctor's condo that also had a lovely view but no light bulb in the bathroom. She was a bit worried that she might bump into something and injure herself again. She had already done it once while being driven home from the doctor's office the morning after her surgery. The driver hit a bump in the road, knocked her out of the seat, and she banged her head and broke a few stitches.

She was somewhat concerned because she was still red as a beet, had a few new pimples on her chin, a wrinkle left under one eye that the doctor had missed (she was going back and have him do it over), and an infection under her ear where the stitches had come undone in her fall in the car.

She wondered vaguely why the doctor didn't provide a nurse's aide or someone in attendance in his $100-a-day condo.

But none of this diminished by one iota her adoration of the doctor. And two weeks later she telephoned me from her home in New Orleans just to let me know that her face looked simply beautiful.

The truth of the matter is, it is almost impossible to find anyone who doesn't think his or her own lifter is a genius.

Curiously, in many years of mingling with the facelift society of Palm Springs I can't offhand recall ever hearing anyone mention the *medical* background of his or her particular lifting genius. People seem more impressed with a lifter's artistic background, his prominence on the social scene, and his Hollywood or VIP connections.

There are thirty doctors listed under "Plastic and Reconstructive Surgery," in the Yellow Pages of the Palm Springs telephone directory. I have checked out most of them, personally interviewed many, and visited their offices, clinics, and recovery facilities, as well as some of their homes.

They are the most fascinating breed of facelifters I have encountered in any city. I call them facelifters as a group rather than plastic surgeons because some are not qualified plastic surgeons even though they list themselves as such in the phone directory.

Many also blatantly advertise their wares under other medical specialty groups, notably with the orthopedic and ENT (Ear-Nose-Throat) specialists.

I doubt if the current social darling of the lift set would be eager to have me for a patient if I went to him with a nosebleed or a broken knee.

Some of the so-called plastic surgeons have longer strung-out lists of specialties than any other doctors in the entire sixteen pages of Physicians and Surgeons.

It must be confusing to anyone who consults the Yellow Pages for an orthopedic or ENT specialist to turn up at the office of a facelifter.

To compound the confusion, some of our top ENT men also do facelifts but are not listed as plastic surgeons.

Some doctors list themselves as "plastic aesthetic" surgeons.

One breaks down his specialties as follows: Breast Implants, Belly Tucks, Facelifts, Acupuncture, Relief Arthritis & Related Problems.

Some carry quarter-page ads with before-and-after pictures.

European-born doctors with exotic names, an aesthetic background, and superior training in the fine arts are more impressive to many clients than medical credentials.

As one of the recent imports told me frankly, "Foreign doctors are more aesthetic than American doctors. Our education is much broader. We understand more about the theater, music, literature, art."

He said he had planned to be an artist or a musician before he went into medicine. He thinks his art training has helped him be a better plastic surgeon because he looks on each face as a painting. His clients love it!

Another artist-lifter has his office walls adorned with his paintings, which evoke rapturous comments: "He's a *real* artist. No wonder he's so good at faces."

Still another of the "plastic aesthetic" surgeons, and one of the social darlings, was very vague and annoyed when I asked him about his medical background but he wasn't at all shy about telling me how he got to be so good at lifting faces.

He said he was born with his artistic talent. His father was a Tyrolean wood sculptor in the Valley of the Dolomites, and passed the art on to him, he said. "As a wood sculptor I learned to appreciate and sculpt beautiful faces, and I still do."

He came to the U.S. at age eighteen, and was a ski instructor and crop duster before going into aesthetic surgery. "I was going into neurosurgery, but I decided there was too much sadness in it," he explained.

"Aesthetic surgery is strictly elective surgery, meaning you need it like a hole in the head, but if it's a luxury you can afford, then you should have the best qualified people to do it. I have earned my reputation because I have limited my practice to faces.

"Who made me what I am?" he asked, quite seriously. "It certainly wasn't doctor referrals. I've done more Hollywood movie stars, more famous people than anyone else around here and I'd been doing them long before these young upstarts moved in.

"Most patients come to me because they've seen my work, they've seen the results, and they know I specialize in faces. I don't do breasts or thighs. I feel that nobody can be good at everything, especially in aesthetic surgery. A face is something so complex that it should not be trusted to someone who also does breasts. Actually, breast augmentation is one of the simplest operations. I have gained a considerable amount of experience and reputation because I limit myself to faces."

A prominent lifter who specializes in all-over bodyworks counters this with, "You can't remain a good doctor and do only faces. A facelift is the least complicated thing to do in aesthetic surgery. A good plastic surgeon is qualified to work on other parts of the body and uses every opportunity to do so. To limit their work to facelifts is a cop-out for those who are not properly qualified and whose aesthetic background is nil."

Apart from their aesthetic expertise, exotic surroundings, and fervent scalpel-swiping, the Palm Springs lifters share a common bond in their enthusiasm for the controversial face peel, which they usually recommend or insist on along with the surgical lift. The peel is more prevalent in Palm Springs than

anywhere else, including Miami, the peel capital. This despite
the fact that peeled faces are supposed to stay out of the sun.

And despite the personal idiosyncrasies of the arty, aesthetic Palm Springs lifters, by and large they continue to turn
out 100-per-cent-satisfied customers. Some have had malpractice suits filed against them. But the percentage is low in ratio
to the number of operations performed. And complaints are
rare except when voiced by an observer who thinks that his or
her particular lift genius could have done a better job.

The Palm Springs social season is a continual round of
parties always scintillating with choice facelift critiques: *She
looks like her ears were pulled off and stuck back on. . . .
You can see the streak around her neck where the peel
stopped. . . . She looks freeze-dried, nothing but cotton between the ears. . . . Something's wrong with her eyes, she
looks like a startled jack rabbit. . . . It's like a new head
screwed onto an old body. . . .*

The most common observation on Palm Springs facelifts,
always noted by outsiders who've had their faces done else-
where, is: "They look as if they all came off an assembly line."

Most lift-watchers agree there is a definite "look" to a
facelift done in Palm Springs. It's known as the hatched in
Palm Springs look; too tight, too tucked, too young, and too
frozen or terrified (it's hard to tell which) to smile.

One of the most popular facelifters, in fact, makes a big
deal of lamenting that his lifted ladies always turn out looking
too young. Like, darn it, he just can't help it if his genius
hands slipped and sculpted a twenty-five-year-old face for an
eighty-year-old body.

Of course this is a sure-fire come-on to aging clients who
scramble through their photo albums for pictures of their lost
youth. He routinely asks prospective facelift candidates, "What
age do you want to look?" They show him pictures and
implore, "Can you make me look like this?" He obligingly
makes a stab at it, often with quite incongruous results; the
new head screwed onto the old body; the hatched in Palm
Springs look with the slit-of-teeth smile.

A friend of mine who recently moved to Palm Springs from New York said that one of the first things she noticed here which intrigued her was the Palm Springs smile. Almost a non-smile.

"A tiny mouth or slit in the face that's too tight to open very far, just enough to show a slit of teeth and then it stops as if frozen. You wonder if she's too tucked up to smile or merely terrified that she'll ruin her facelift if she smiles and have to have it done over again. The thing I miss most around here," she said, "is an honest-to-God, ear-to-ear smile."

Actually, the main reason for the too-tight, mask-like, hatched in Palm Springs facelift is that many of the faces have already been done many times before.

There is absolutely no reason for your facelift to have a tight, mask-like appearance if you choose the right doctor and use common sense in your individual needs instead of playing Follow the Leader.

Because I happen to live in Palm Springs I frequently get calls from people in distant places asking me to recommend a facelifter.

I do not personally recommend or endorse any doctor to do your facelift. And let me make clear that it is not the intention of this book to make recommendations, so you can save yourselves the phone calls and postage stamps.

As stated in my preface, the purpose of this book is to give a second opinion, based on well-researched facts and personal experience, to help *you* decide whether you want a facelift or not.

Palm Springs happens to be one of the front-runners in the facelifting Olympics, and a lot of people are pointing their faces in this direction.

Most of the lifted faces I've seen turn out okay whether they're done by Dr. W, X, Y, or Z. Or ENT.

It's mostly a matter of personal preference and prejudice. If you can't stand camels and llamas, for instance, you can opt for the lifter with his goat-and-horse recovery ranch.

You may prefer the self-proclaimed King of Plastic Surgery in his cowboy boots and gold-studded jumpsuits or the Dr. Little Lord Fauntleroy with his boyish blow-dry hairdo and indoor waterfall.

One thing is certain: nowhere else will you get such exotic fringe benefits with your facelift as you will in Palm Springs.

You may even bump into Lucille Ball or Natalie Wood in I. Magnin's.

And it's for sure you're going to see one of the Gabors. You can't miss them.

As this was written, Magda, the eldest of the Gabor sisters and in my opinion the most beautiful, had just had her face done again, this time by the doctor who did such a sensational job on Mama Jolie. The day after her surgery, Magda was driven to her mansion in the foothills of the San Jacinto mountains only to be greeted by a squadron of fire engines and a large crew of fire fighters trying to control a mountain blaze that was raging within yards of her home.

The firemen tried to prevent her from entering the house. She marched in and refused to be evacuated.

Her new face was still in bandages and even her beau couldn't budge her out of the house. She wasn't taking any chances on doing anything to mess up her new facelift, she said —except risk her life for it.

P.S. The fire was brought under control and Magda's new face looks sensational!

Considering the kookiness of the lifestyle in Palm Springs and the total dedication to one-upmanship among the beauty and youth cults, the wonder is that so many facelifts turn out as well as they do.

Why have your face done in Omaha when you can have it done in a glamorous and glittering movieland setting?

It is exactly this that attracts thousands of youth seekers to both Palm Springs and Los Angeles, which has always considered itself the plastic surgery capital of the world. Los Angeles, of course, has its own self-proclaimed King of Plastic Surgery, who also wears cowboy boots and gold-studded jumpsuits.

It's simply taken for granted that in the Tinseltown precincts of Southern California, plastic surgery is merely an adjunct of the beauty industry and has more in common with the hairdressing salon than with the medical profession.

The truth is, your face doctors in Omaha, Memphis, or Tallahassee probably have just as good medical credentials as those in Palm Springs or Beverly Hills.

And the truth is, there may be quite a few bona fide, super-qualified cosmetic surgeons out here who keep a low profile and do fine work without throwing in all the exotic fringe benefits. It's just harder to find them among all the Hollywood hype and trappings.

However, the same is true in all branches of medicine as in all branches of anything else in this state of shimmering stardust and moonbeams.

My personal advice to anyone who is giving thoughtful consideration to having a facelift is to think twice about it before buying your plane ticket to *anywhere* in Southern California.

Don't get me wrong. I live here. I love it. And some of my best friends are doctors. But if I'm going to have my face done, I would be wary of Tyrolean wood carvers playing the movie game. I would prefer to check out their medical credentials rather than their camels, llamas, or skewered shish kebab.

As I've noted, the majority of people who come here for their facelifts have already been to other places, other facelifters. They come here for the movieland fun-and-games and because it's fashionable, the *in* place for the Beautiful People set.

For those of you who have not yet had your *first* facelift, I strongly recommend that you reread this chapter carefully and if you should decide on a Tinseltown lift, be sure to check and double-check, then triple-check the doctor's qualifications and look at the results of his work.

Your face most likely will turn out fine if you can afford to follow the Beautiful People wherever they go.

But there are other places and other facelifters also turning out 100-per-cent-satisfied customers.

4

Pygmalion of Papeete

Whoever heard of going to Tahiti for a facelift?

A lot of people.

Dr. Jean-Paul Lintilhac, a transplanted Pygmalion from Paris, is the new superstar of plastic surgery for the Beautiful People who prefer going to exotic foreign places for their lifts.

His posh facelift salon and rejuvenation clinic in the heart of downtown Papeete is stealing a lot of the sags, bags, and bodyworks business away from Rio's Dr. Ivo Pitanguy (pronounced Pee-tang-ee), known to one and all as "dear Ivo," who for years reigned as the international, socialite superstar of plastic surgeons. Dear Ivo is most famous for bottoms, bellies, and breast reduction.

Until recently all the chic people were making the Rio connection for the "Pitanguy Look" in everything from nose bobs to trimmed derrières. Now they're making the pilgrimage to Papeete for the "Lintilhac Lift," performed by a darkly handsome, barely sixtyish plastic surgeon whose clinics in Cannes and Paris were popular with the French Riviera social set as well as some of Europe's top film beauties.

He moved to Tahiti (which is French) only a few years ago and many of his clients have followed him.

Society columnist Suzy Knickerbocker once accorded Dr. Lintilhac superstar status on her personal-recommendation list of eight of the world's top plastic surgeons to the Beautiful People.

(The others were: Rio's Dr. Pitanguy; London's Dr. Robin Beare; New York's Drs. David Ju, Thomas Rees, John Converse (recently deceased); Miami's Dr. Ralph Millard; and Dr. Franklyn Ashley of Beverly Hills, who did Phyllis Diller's face and many more of the movie stars.)

The coconut grapevine, which operates as a news media with astonishing speed and accuracy throughout the South Sea Islands (far superior to U.S. gossip columns), reports that Sophia Loren and Catherine Deneuve have been spotted going in or out of the Lintilhac Salon.

I asked Dr. Lintilhac about these rumors when I visited his salon. He replied discreetly in soft-spoken, near-perfect English, "I do not discuss with anyone my patients."

But it's unlikely that they jet to Tahiti just to see Marlon Brando.

Unlike some BP plastic surgeons who ply their trade with flamboyance and no lack of reticence in blowing their own horns, Dr. Lintilhac is very low profile, an unpompous, scholarly, quietly reserved man of few words and exquisite aesthetic tastes.

His perennial Exhibit A is Simone Lintilhac, his wife of nearly thirty years, who still looks as young and beautiful as she did at twenty-five when he married her.

"I am keeping her the way I want her to be. Why not? She is my wife," he says proudly.

He's done her face twice, and everything else—almost.

"Here and here and here, all over, everywhere," Simone says, gracefully patting her face and fanny, eyes, thighs, tummy, and chest.

In a lyrical mélange of groping English and French, she admits with disarming candor, "I am fifty-four. My husband, he ees very *artiste*, non? *Oui*. I close my eyes and say, 'Operate me.' *Voilà!*"

Voilà! At fifty-four, Simone is a dazzling walking testimonial for the Lintilhac Lift in all of its varied anatomical locations. The only untouched appendage is her nose.

"Her nose doesn't need changing," says Dr. Lintilhac. "It's fine the way it is. Besides, we have more problems psychologically with noses."

Ironically, since moving to Tahiti he's had a booming business in nose bobs—from natives who want a nose like Simone's.

While it's the trendy thing for many plastic surgeons to marry their ladies, make them over, and then turn them in for a new model, Dr. Lintilhac is content with his resculptured original. Her two facelifts and assorted body-contouring jobs have transformed her into one of those sylph-like visions of beauty and eternal youth that most women would die for.

But before all of you start hopping the next plane to Tahiti, let me warn you: Don't expect to come back looking like Simone. She had a lot going for her in the first place. She was a former fashion model in Paris, and her natural endowments required minimal remolding.

But she believes in having a little tuck here and there as needed, and with a live-in snip-and-stitch artist to do it, why not? She doesn't have to go through the dreadful dilemma that most women must wrestle with: How to choose a doctor.

Simone is the first to tell you, quite frankly, that her husband is a genius. A man of extraordinary modesty for the type of business he's in, he disclaims any special prowess with the scalpel and makes no grandiose claims to either medical or artistic super-talents. He is, in fact, refreshingly the exact antithesis of the Hollywood-hype type lifter.

Moreover, his medical credentials and international reputation with his peers are all in top-drawer shape; he doesn't need to toss in exotica or braggadocio to get clients. Though born in Bordeaux, most of his medical training was in London and New York. He was widely recognized for his work in reconstructive plastic surgery during World War II and has written extensively on cosmetic surgery, in books and scientific papers for medical journals.

His clinics in Paris and Cannes were virtual shrines of the international Beautiful People jet-setters always in search of a lift. Because of the demands on his time he gave up his practice and moved to Tahiti, intending to take it easy with an early "retirement"—which came to an abrupt end as soon as the coconut grapevine wafted word across the Pacific as to his whereabouts.

Voilà! Came the stampede. His devotees, no doubt bored with going to the same old places for their new faces, welcomed his relocation in the heavenly South Seas.

In fact, the medical trek to Tahiti for a facelift has its own built-in fringe benefits, which rival those anywhere in the world: nubile Polynesian vahines in slithering pareaus hanging garlands of fragrant frangipani around your neck; post-operative care and pampering in beautiful beachfront hotels, with Tahitian dancers in pandanus skirts to entertain you; island hops to Huahiné, Moorea, and Bora-Bora—the one James Michener once described as the most beautiful island in the world. And it still is. Booming tourism has barely touched the primitive, enchanting beauty of these islands, in spite of what the iconoclasts say.

The first question most people have asked me about Tahiti is, "But what are the medical facilities like?"

As I mentioned earlier, I have rarely been asked about the medical qualifications—or medical facilities—of any facelifter in the United States, but for some reason many people assume there are no modern medical facilities in Tahiti.

Dr. Lintilhac and his staff operate in one of the most modern and impressive cosmetic surgery centers I have seen anywhere. It is a five-story building officially designated as the South Pacific Cosmedical Center but commonly referred to as the Lintilhac Clinic. This is a misnomer. It's more like a salon.

The top floor contains the surgical arena with a reception-waiting room as swank as any bordering the *Bois de Bologne* and an operating room so antiseptic that it could be used for open-heart surgery.

Private clinics for cosmetic surgery are sometimes described as "mini-hospitals." In this case, another misnomer. For here there is none of the familiar clattering and odoriferous aura of either clinic or hospital.

Yet it has all the necessary medical securities and guarantees, some of which do not even exist in the best hospitals.

For example, an anesthesia machine (RPR) which is reputedly the most modern and sophisticated type made—and an anesthesiologist experienced in long and serious operations in one of the best hospitals in France, now working under contract exclusively for the Lintilhac Clinic.

To qualify for a Lintilhac Lift you must have a complete medical checkup (though the doctor's surgery never touches a vital organ); then your face and body will be examined from an aesthetic viewpoint by a beautification team—plastic surgeon, oral surgeon, and dermatologist.

Dr. Lintilhac does his facelifts in two separate operations, the face first, eyes the next day. (About two and a half to three hours for the facelift, or rhytidectomy; one and a half hours for the eyelift, or blepharoplasty). Many women want only their eyes done but he very seldom does eyes alone. "You shouldn't do eyes without the facelift," he says.

Patients spend two nights in the clinic, then ten days to two weeks of post-operative care in a hotel.

The facelift fee in Tahiti is about half what you would pay in most U.S. cities. But there is also your round-trip air fare to consider, approximately $800 from Los Angeles, and your $100-a-day beachfront bungalow for recuperation.

Dr. Lintilhac recommends that patients remain in Papeete for two weeks after surgery. That isn't too hard to take. The view of Moorea when your baggy eyelids have been lifted is truly one of the most spectacular views in the world.

Cosmetic surgery is only one part of Dr. Lintilhac's total rejuvenation program.

"Looking young is *almost* being young, but not quite," he says. "Cosmetic surgery is fine for the outside but you must do something for the inside too."

What he is doing for the inside is a rather mind-boggling

adaptation of practically all the youth-giving or youth-preservation treatments, techniques, shots, therapies, and medical and mechanical aids ever conceived.

You can get anything from acupuncture to procaine for your health, beauty, and youth problems; plus whirlpool baths in imported giant tubs with gold-plated faucets and spurting fountains, guaranteed to make you lose weight. While I was there, I talked to a man from Minneapolis who swore he had lost two pounds in half an hour.

All of this non-surgical but medically supervised rejuvenation is programmed on the other four floors of the clinic.

Actually the clinic—or salon—is rather like an ultra-posh, perpendicular spa combining the best of Elizabeth Arden's Maine Chance and California's Golden Door, and with the "mini-hospital" or surgical arena at the top.

Among the many rejuvenation therapies he uses are the renowned "youth shots" of Switzerland, an adaptation of the Niehans cellular therapy from sheep embryos, still frowned on by the AMA but much sought after by the rich and famous and young at heart.

It's hard to imagine the predicament Ponce de León would have been in if faced with so many Fountain-of-Youth options under one roof.

Dr. Lintilhac admits that he created the options as much for himself as anyone else.

"A plastic surgeon, any surgeon, knows that the time will come when he must give up the scalpel. As a cosmetic surgeon I have loved my work and I believe in it. When I can no longer operate on others," he said, "perhaps I will have time to extend my own youth. A little."

Before leaving I overheard a woman ask him wistfully, "Do you think you could make me look like Simone?"

"No more than I could look like Robert Redford," he replied seriously. "A facelift isn't a miracle. It's merely an improvement on what nature gave you."

5

Which Lady Has the Lift?

(Do You Really Need It?)

I've already warned you that you'll need to do a lot of soul-searching in trying to decide Should I? Or Shouldn't I?

Most doctors will tell you that if you're going to have a facelift it should be done when you're in your forties instead of waiting until you're sixty. Most of the facelifted women I've talked to don't pay too much attention to what the doctors tell them on this score (as well as others); many have lifts in their thirties, and in their seventies and eighties.

In nearly every medical book or article on the subject, you'll find the question: *What is the ideal age for facial surgery?* The answers vary among doctors who dwell on psychological motivations. The best answer comes from the patients themselves, who almost in unison say, "The age to have it done is when you need it." Though a good many advise, "You should have it done *before* you think you need it." What they really mean is—before *others* think you need it, before that first wee wrinkle grows into full-blown crow's feet.

The truth is, there is no "ideal" age for a facelift since no two people conform to the chronological aging process in exactly the same way, except possibly identical twins; and even they might not age at the same wrinkle rate if, for instance, one smokes, drinks, and fries in the sun and the other doesn't.

Whether and when you need a facelift depends on many factors: heredity and environment, your bone structure, skin texture, and lifestyle; your personal habits, disciplines, desires, and practical problems; your genes and genealogy as well as your *joie de vivre;* the twinkle in your eye as well as your underskin fat.

All of these add up to wrinkles, no wrinkles, or more wrinkles, and I've seen many forty-five-year-old wrinkled-prune faces that look more like fifty-five or sixty. (If you're one of these, I'd say you definitely need a lift, but that's up to you.)

I've also seen seventy-plus women with lifted faces that could pass for twenty-five to thirty.

In considering whether to have a facelift, you're going to run into a lot of medical exhortations about "realistic expectations" such as: You can't turn back the clock; you should not expect to look younger, only better.

Anyone who tells you that is off his rocker. I've seen hundreds of lifted faces that look ten, twenty, even thirty and forty years younger than their chronological age. I'm not saying they look better, but they do look younger. I'm talking only of faces. In fact I've seen some so facelifted that I almost didn't recognize them from one party to the next. And some of them, I might add, look rather ridiculous with a thirtyish face jutting out from a septuagenarian shoulder hump and shriveled neck.

How much better you'll look when you're de-aged depends a great deal on the shape you're in from the chin down.

What causes skin aging—changing—wearing out?

The medical consensus:

• Tissues wear out, just from time, and just as a machine wears out. But the aging process is variable according to skin types, pigmentation, elasticity, stress and strain, weight loss, and so on.

• Skin is stretchable and can be pulled out of shape, even while you sleep. You should never sleep on your side in curlicue fashion; nor ostrich-style with your head buried in pillows; nor lying on your stomach face down—all of this is just asking for wrinkles and creases and crow's feet in your face and neck, torso, arms, legs, fingers, and toes, we're told. This doesn't leave us much choice, does it?

The correct way to slumber is flat on your back, relaxed, legs spread apart, arms stretched and raised toward your head, and a tiny pillow under your neck. And for heaven's sake, don't hug it!

Quotes from Experts:

• Dr. A. . . . "Skin does not expand in volume; it is constantly growing but sloughing off as cells die."

• Dr. B. . . . "Facial skin does not grow, but it never ceases to age. No one can stop the normal aging process of the skin."

• Dr. C. . . . "The aging process can be reversed or slowed by . . ." etcetera.

• Dr. D. . . . "Think of your face as a rubber band. Every time you laugh, cry, frown, eat, drink, smoke, or kiss, you stretch that rubber band. When you go outdoors, you bake it in the sun, freeze it in the snow, or dry it in the wind. Any wonder that the rubber band gives?"

It's asking a lot of any woman to give up all these things for a tight rubber-band face. Most of them prefer to go on at least kissing and living and taking their chances. An interesting paradox is that some women can look as young and beautiful at fifty-four *without* a facelift as others the same age with several lifts.

There is Simone Lintilhac, for example, mentioned in the previous chapter. With her husband's help she still looks very much like the twenty-five-year-old Paris model he married and molded into what he still wants her to look like at fifty-four.

But I know women as wrinkle-free, youthful, and beautiful as Simone at the same age, and *without* a facelift—and so do you. Stack them up together; ask which one has the lift? (Like, which one has the Toni?) You can't tell the difference.

Simone has done everything right, according to the rules. She doesn't smoke, drink, or bake in the sun. Lady X has done everything wrong: she smokes, drinks, sunbathes daily, and sleeps ostrich-like with her head buried in pillows. Yet her unlifted face is as wrinkle-free as Simone's twice-lifted one.

How can there be such an aging discrepancy? How can a fifty-four-year-old woman without a facelift look as good as a fifty-four-year-old woman with a couple or more?

In the case of Lady X it's mostly a matter of being born with high wall-to-wall cheekbones, and then taking care of them. She learned the hard way—by getting a severe sunburn when she was only eighteen. She fell asleep for hours on the beach. "It was one of the luckiest things that ever happened to me," she says, "because I suddenly knew inside of me that I would never in my life go out in the sun again with naked skin." Since then taking care of her skin has become almost a fetish with her, and it has paid off—she looks . . . well . . . not too bad for fifty-four without a lift.

When I compare the overretouched women I've met with those who haven't been retouched at all, I think of my friend Dodie Foote, who at seventy-one looks fifteen to twenty years younger and is still lithe, vibrant, attractive, and remarkably unlined for her age. How come?

Her doting husband Doc has his own answer: "She's loved dearly."

Doc is William A. Foote, famous painter of clowns. He is seventy-six years young and his influence may indeed have a lot to do with his wife's youthfulness. He still treats her like a child bride. We should all be so lucky! "I've taught her how to feel secure in the present and not to worry about the future," he says. Their "statement" of life is reflected not only in their happy faces but in their twinkling eyes and rippling laughter and exuberance for living. Both are artists, but both have captured an art of living that has nothing to do with chronological age. Instead of wall-to-wall cheekbones they have wall-to-wall clown paintings to hold up their rubber-band bounce.

Says Dodie, "It's all in the way you *think*. I've always *thought* right. I think the thought processes have so much to do with the way we look and the way we get old. It may sound child-like but I do not permit myself the privilege of dwelling on something that hurts or is painful. It's like if my finger gets caught in a door—sure, it hurts, but I keep saying it doesn't hurt and then it doesn't.

"Sure, I get upset, that's the human equation, but I think you can control your emotional upsets if you think right. And you won't have so many headaches or wrinkles."

Has Dodie ever considered a facelift?

"I could stand one," she chuckles, "but what if I paid $5,000 for a facelift and dropped dead tomorrow? At my age it isn't that important. I think too many people are obsessed with self-image for others to look at. I'm happy with being just me."

Many women will identify with Dodie. But if you don't have happy thoughts or wall-to-wall cheekbones, you may need a facelift and the time to do it is when you want it. The ideal age is when you look in the mirror and say to yourself, "Hey, those aren't character lines, they're creases from sleeping scrunched up in the pillows."

6

Darling, I'm Dripping...

I Want a Facelift from the Ankles Up . . .

Why do you want a facelift?

Do you want it to hold a husband or a job?

What is your "psychological motivation" for wanting a facelift?

Most doctors—not all—say this is very important. I say it's baloney and hogwash. So do most patients and a few of the more honest doctors.

Many women are intimidated into guilt feelings about even wanting a facelift by the widespread propaganda of plastic surgeons who pompously proclaim self-anointed psychoanalytic prowess along with their surgical scalpel.

Some doctors claim to refuse about one third of their applicants, emphasizing the fact that they take great pains to examine the "psychological factors" involved in someone's seeking cosmetic surgery.

So far I've never met anyone who has even been asked about their "psychological factors," much less rejected for them, though I know a few who have been refused for medical reasons (lung cancer).

The psychological motivation of most women boils down to a simple common denominator—they want it.

In the words of a friend of mine frequently expressed to her husband, "Darling, I'm dripping. I want a facelift from the ankles up."

And that's a good enough reason for her. She's not husband- or job-shopping. She has no Freudian motive that she knows of, no id or ego problem or Oedipus complex; she simply wishes now and then, as most women do, that she could have a few lifts here and there; and when she decides to do it, if a doctor has the audacity to ask her *why,* she'll tell him it's none of his business.

So would I.

One of the nation's most highly esteemed plastic surgeons told me, "Most of our patients have very strong psychological problems. We're dealing with a more psychiatrically—I hate to use the term 'abnormal' because I don't think there is anything that's normal—but we're dealing with patients with more neuroticism than in the general population, let's say. That's why they're here. I'm not saying that people who come in for facelifts are *nuts*, but they are different from the so-called normal population."

So okay, we're nuts.

But the doctor adds, "Curiously enough, the psychiatrists are absolutely baffled by us, because 98 per cent of our patients do very well with facelifts."

Just between us nuts it will be fascinating to watch the facelifters put the head-shrinkers out of business.

On a saner level there are some dissenting opinions on the importance of probing your psyche to find out *why* you want a facelift.

"Pompous nonsense and presumptuous," Dr. Jean-Paul Lintilhac says of the self-styled psychoanalysts prevalent in cosmetic surgery, who are trying to excavate hidden motivations or some deep-seated neurosis that might trigger your desire for a facelift.

"Psychological motivation isn't the domain of plastic surgeons. We are unqualified by training and temperament to pass judgment on a patient's motivation for cosmetic surgery. Yet, some want to appear as doctors of the mind. I think they're motivated for more deep-seated psychological reasons than their patients.

"My own psychoanalytical theory"—he says it with a smile—"is that cosmetic surgery is a specialty that removes the inferiority complex of the patients and gives it to the surgeons.

"They develop guilt feelings about using their skills only to beautify the body," he explained, "and so attempt to justify it with a psychological cross-examination: Is this operation necessary? If so, why?

"It's not really our business to ask why. Most people have their minds made up before they come to a plastic surgeon. Maybe they've already been to a marriage counselor or a divorce lawyer; their husbands are playing around or they're trying to find a new husband. They know a facelift will make them look better and feel younger. I know it too. I am qualified only as a plastic surgeon, not as a psychiatrist or psychological counselor.

"Of course," he added, "we must be careful. I try to eliminate the real nuts. But sometimes I waste more time trying to throw them out than I would spend on a facelift, so I figure I might as well do a little for them."

Dr. B. G. Gross, dermatologist at the Derma-Lift Salon in Miami (widely known for its chemosurgical facelifts), is equally emphatic: "I think it is presumptuous for a dermatologist or a plastic surgeon to make a psychological judgment on a patient who comes in for a facelift. We are absolutely unqualified by training and temperament to pass judgment on the whys and wherefores; that is not our business. Our patients have to pass a thorough physical examination before we take them but we don't give them mental aptitude tests. Sure, we get some kooks, who doesn't? But they're in the minority and we handle them. We do facelifts, we're not psychologists, we don't ask about their so-called motivations. It's pompous nonsense."

Dr. Bengt Nylen, head of the Department of Plastic Surgery at Karolinska Hospital and professor at the University of Stockholm, Sweden, says, "I don't ask the patients why they want it done. If I were a psychiatrist, I perhaps could find out the real reason. But if they're sound, healthy, and if their motivations seem to be sound and their face corresponds to their complaints, I think it should be done."

For some strange reason, plastic surgeons in New York seem to be more psyched out on the motivational syndrome than those in other cities. Some also expressed doubts about my qualifications to interview them since I do not have a medical degree and they took a dim view of my ability to interpret their remarks properly.

I have my own doubts about a doctor's qualifications to do in-depth probing of facelift patients' psychological needs if the doctor does not have a degree in psychology or psychiatry, and I take a dim view of his ability to interpret properly whether a patient is deeply disturbed, schizophrenic, or any more nuts than he is.

Following is the verbatim statement of a top New York plastic surgeon from his taped interview: "The surgeon has to be confident of the motives of the patient. Some are able to conceal deeply disturbing psychological conditions, even schizophrenia." How does *he* know? "Probing interviews and experience will help reveal such situations, which are fraught with risks for both the surgeon and the patient."

Another, a relative newcomer to New York with one of those arty-European backgrounds, refused to be interviewed but gave me his "curriculum vitae," which, if I interpret it properly, indicates he is also a newcomer to plastic surgery with some unique qualifications including, in addition to his medical training, a degree in marine biology, a course in opera at the Academy of Music in Paris, and "instinctive abilities" in the area of plastic surgery.

"Due to the advantageous combination of European and American surgical experience," his puff sheet reads, "the Doctor has developed his own individual approach to various plastic surgical procedures, which includes an in-depth awareness of the patient's psychological needs. The Doctor feels this is an essential entity in order to achieve the best possible result."

Whether the Doctor derived his in-depth awareness of psychological matters from his study of marine biology and opera or through ESP, it's difficult to guess. With his "instinctive abilities" he may do the greatest face jobs in the world (though I doubt it), but if you need your psyche analyzed, you should take it to a psychiatrist, not a facelifter.

Another plastic surgeon warns in cutesy nonsense: "A facelift cannot change the psyche, it merely alters the façade."

Everyone knows that when you look better, you feel better, which is the same as changing the "psyche." Even most doctors agree on this.

A top plastic surgeon in Chicago puts it this way: "I think most patients today are realistic enough to know that we don't make any promises or guarantees that we will make them look X number of years younger; we strive to make them look better and if in the process they also look younger, that's fine. Often people do look younger when you make them look better; and then they *feel* better too."

Of course there are patients who sometimes pose obvious psychological problems to plastic surgeons who should and usually do recognize them without in-depth psychoanalytical probing. Some doctors turn down these patients; others take a chance on them. Betty Ford is the most famous case in point. As mentioned earlier, some doctors felt she should not have had a facelift so soon after her drug and alcohol rehabilitation. Many doctors refuse to take patients who are overweight—or they'll postpone the lift until the patient loses weight. And meanwhile a lot of patients simply go out shopping for another doctor who doesn't mind if they're obese. I've seen quite a few lifted ladies who would have looked better if they had spent their time and money in a spa for reducing pounds instead of wrinkles. p

I've also heard of doctors who claim to refuse patients whose type of face doesn't lend itself to good results—or to results that will please the patient. There are no doubt a number of good and valid reasons for doctors to turn down patients for cosmetic surgery. No doctor in his right mind, for instance, wants to take on a drug addict or real psycho if he can help it. If a patient is going through a personal crisis, it might not be a wise time for a facelift; or it could be a good time. A widow who is still grieving over the death of her husband after six months, for example, might be helped over her depression with a facelift. Or she might not. The competent, experienced plastic surgeon should have enough common horse-sense psychology and rapport with his patients to be able to recognize red-light danger signals; and he should be able to screen patients carefully, if he really wants to, without playing the role of a mind doctor.

On the other hand, the patients themselves should give it more serious thought.

As one plastic surgeon told me, "Some people come in thinking it's something to have done on your lunch hour. It isn't; it's a major procedure. To do this without giving thought to it, for frivolous reasons, is very unwise."

I agree wholeheartedly, which is the reason for this book.

However, I feel that the overemphasis on psychological motivation has itself contributed to psychological problems for patients, many of whom feel embarrassed or guilty at even asking for a facelift, and too self-conscious about vanity.

What's wrong with vanity? Isn't it related to self-respect?

What's wrong with a woman wanting a facelift for no ulterior motive, for no other reason than that she wants to look better?

Maybe she's the type who finds the signs of age discouraging; she feels young and vital, but looks older than she feels.

Even some doctors agree that it's all right for us to want to look better and we don't need any other motivation for a facelift. Says one: "The reason for cosmetic surgery is that we feel better if we think we look better."

Says another: "People do it for themselves because they

want to look better, because they want to look younger. It's pride in one's self, which is different from sheer vanity."

Phyllis Diller's comment: "It isn't a sin to look better."

And even Ann Landers, whose advice tends to be on the conservative side—she's often been called a "square"—has this to say: "I have received many letters from readers wanting to know about facelifts and I tell them all—If a facelift will make you feel better about yourself, go ahead and do it!"

My own advice: Darlings, if you're dripping—or drooping —and want a facelift from the ankles up, steer clear of the lifters who want to analyze your psyche.

7

Come Out of the Closets, Male Peacocks . . .

Women's lib has done a lot for men too, but apart from some young dudes who've had their faces redone to look like Elvis Presley, the men are Mickey Mouses when it comes to admitting they've had a facelift.

As one top plastic surgeon told me, "For some reason, men feel more guilty about it than women. I don't know why."

One theory is that men once looked on the facelift as unmasculine and some perhaps still do. But the evidence strongly indicates that this outlook is rapidly changing and that men are at last losing their inhibitions in the vanity marathon.

There has never been any question that men basically are more vain than women. Historically, men have always been the buttons-and-bows type, with their ruffles and wigs, all powdered and plumed like strutting peacocks. In the literature of plastic surgery you'll find some rather astonishing examples of men's vigorous efforts to retain or regain their virility and youth. Some really used their imagination to look younger. France's Cardinal Richelieu, for instance, was known to pull back his hair tightly from the temples so that it would stretch the skin around his eyes and hide the wrinkles.

For many years facelifts for men represented only about 5 per cent of the plastic surgeon's business, and most of these were for movie stars or others in the public eye. Men now make up about 25 per cent of the lift business and they include every conceivable working category from truck drivers to pilots, business executives, teachers, politicians, and many retired senior citizens.

Men were once so terribly shy and guilt-ridden about having a facelift that they usually ran off to Rio to have it done. No more. A New York plastic surgeon reports that about half his patients are men. And in Beverly Hills, where everyone boasts the biggest, the best, or the most, one of the top bananas told me frankly, "I do more men than anyone in the country. I love doing men. They're a little fussy but they will settle for a little bit less than women. And they're a lot more grateful."

One of his patients was forty-eight years old and when the facelifter finished with him—well, let him tell it:

"Every time he goes into a bar, they ask him for his ID card. And he's now doing well over a million dollars' worth of business a year for his company. He's a young, vigorous salesman with an up-and-coming company and he's made a great deal of money from his facelift. He says, 'Now they look at me and know I'm young.' His facelift has paid off over and above a thousand times what it cost him.

"He's a special case, very unusual. I get quite a few men who want a lift because they're in a competitive business but I also get a lot for sheer vanity reasons—because they're still chasing around. One of my patients has a neck problem which runs in the family. I keep doing his neck every time he's chasing a new girl friend. I have another one, about sixty-five, who still plays tennis every day and he's now on his third wife. The last time he came in, he wanted just enough [of a lift] to go along with his new wife, so he wouldn't look too much older.

He's had a hair transplant too, but that didn't turn out too well . . ."

And incidentally, this doctor told me he sometimes does his facelifts under hypnosis instead of more orthodox forms of anesthesia.

In today's youth-conscious society, with more and more people concerned about their image, women's lib seems to have caused an identity crisis for men, who also are being liberated in their own self-beautification boom.

"It's the ERA in reverse," one expert said, pointing out that male chauvinists are stealing the thunder right out from under milady's vanity table.

Crystal-gazers predict that by the year 2000 men will be using most of the beauty items that women use today.

Already that national institution known as the beauty salon, once strictly a ladies-only emporium, has switched gears to accommodate Mr. Average-Man-on-the-Street (from restaurateurs to CPAs), who comes in for a new perm or touch-up, a color job or curling-iron wave, a manicure, pedicure, facial, eyebrow tint, wig set or reshaping of his hairpiece—all the things women do, plus some more.

In their quest for youth and beauty, growing numbers of "average" men are about to overtake the women in getting rid of their sags and bags, seeking facelifts, nose bobs, eye jobs, and related cosmetic procedures to remove the ravages of age, improve job prospects, and enhance their looks.

As for generalities, here are a few startling statistics: $90 million per year for mouthwash and gargles (mostly for men); $500 million a year business in wigs, toupees, more elegantly called hairpieces for men; $10,000-per-head hair transplants, now as *in* as heart transplants; a multimillion-dollar business in men's perfumes, jewelry, chains, and etceteras; and more millions for everyone—specialists—from body-watchers to facelifters; men's boutiques abound and special men's beauty salons in top name beauticians' and cosmetologists' once-for-women havens now cater to male personages such as Tiny Tim and Cary Grant.

At my own beauty shop in Palm Springs, men and women sit alongside one another at mirrors and manicure tables; at least a third of the business is men; some days there are more men than women in the shop. Recently a big burly truck-driver type came in with his wife(?), who sat and waited for *him* while he got a shampoo, set, and manicure. A real role switch. And not long ago at the San Diego airport I saw a *man* wandering around with his hair done up in big fat pink rollers yet! And wearing a hair net. Like those female slobs in supermarkets.

As a cosmetologist who caters to the male beauty trade said, "So they're finally liberated and they're stealing all these feminine things to make them mucho-macho—from permanent waves to silk bikinis. The only thing they're not doing that women do is the false eyelashes."

In the lifting department they're outdoing women in some anatomical areas. The newest wrinkle in the male sags-and-bags armamentarium is the penis-lift.

This of course is *sub rosa* and not the type of thing you consult your friendly family physician about.

There's also a run on chin dimples. Many men think that dimples are attractive and request that distinctive depression in the center of their chins to help make them as sexy, they hope, as Cary Grant or Kirk Douglas.

There are also reports that one big male star has had a dimple lift.

Chin dimples, incidentally, are generally a family characteristic, but cosmetic surgeons, besieged with requests to create artificial ones, have perfected the knack of carving a notch in the center of a chin implant that is a reasonably good facsimile of a dimple. However, handmade dimples, the experts warn, are often not exactly centered, symmetrical, or natural in appearance and they do not move as the face moves. Patients who insist on the chin dimple are willing to take this risk—the same as they do with the facelift, which often leaves one eye bigger than the other and the face not exactly symmetrical.

Another indication of the increase in cosmetic surgery for men was a recent report from a government agency, the Department of Health, Education and Welfare, which revealed that cosmetic surgery for military personnel is costing taxpayers up to $6 million a year.

The report said that surgeons are providing about 3,000 patients each year with free facelifts and other "beauty operations." The statistics were based on an investigation of the records of military and Public Health Service hospitals nationwide.

"My jowls were beginning to sag," said a retired colonel, who told a reporter he had his wrinkles flattened in the public health hospital in San Francisco. "I needed a new image."

Records at this one public health hospital in San Francisco showed that its plastic surgeon had performed 1,110 nose jobs, facelifts, and "other beauty treatments" in the four years (1973–77) before he went into private practice.

Military and public health hospital systems offer cosmetic surgery as part of the free medical services for military personnel in uniform or retired, and their dependents. But an investigation of surgery in Public Health Service hospitals has been launched because, as Joseph Califano, former secretary of the Department of Health, Education and Welfare, said, "I doubt that we should be in the business of non-therapeutic facelifts."

Generally, men do not show their age as much as women do. At the same age a woman will look older than a man because her skin is thinner. Some doctors say that the daily ritual of shaving, which involves a certain amount of massaging and toning, helps preserve the elasticity of the male's facial skin. Also, because of the hair follicles in the beard, even after shaving, the skin is thicker and so the wrinkles, the jowls, and bags don't show through.

However, there are always exceptions to the generalities. A jet airline pilot admitted he was bugged at the way passengers sometimes looked at him, as though thinking, "Is that old man the pilot? What if he has a heart attack?" He was only in his early fifties, tall, slim, and athletic, and in exceptionally good physical shape even for a man twenty years younger. All airline pilots are required to pass rigorous physical fitness tests and there was no doubt about the jet pilot's fitness.

"But I have almost white hair, and recently I had started to sag a bit at the jowls and under the eyes," he said. "I suppose it's just that I'm that type." So he flew to Rio for a "vacation" and went back to work with a younger, leaner-looking face.

It is generally agreed that the growing number of men resorting to cosmetic surgery is part of the over-all picture of its greater acceptance by society. But in many cases, to be sure, there is more than male vanity involved. As one plastic surgeon puts it:

"One of the reasons driving men to have facelifts is competition for jobs in a technological world in which the accent is on young men with skills in the latest techniques. There are some men whose facial skin stretches and sags, no matter how well they take care of their physical condition. They keep fit, live a healthy life, have a sensible diet, buy good clothes, and keep themselves well groomed. Their appearance is important. In most cases there are no problems about their ability to do the job—but it's the younger men who get the promotions."

Employment experts agree that it is more difficult for older men to get promotions or to find work because of the increasing number of competent young men.

Most cosmetic surgeons can cite numerous cases of men who got other jobs in the same business after having a facelift. There is even one case of a man who was fired, had a facelift, and later fought his way back into his old job. Such cases are probably rare.

An interesting sidelight on the occupational hazards of aging—or permitting your age to show—is a report that the Russians provide cosmetic surgery as part of their workers' benefits.

The quest for the illusion of youth and beauty isn't confined only to American society. At plastic surgeons' conferences in other world centers, leading surgeons from many countries have commented especially on the rapidly rising percentage of their male patients.

In the United States, doctors also have noted a significant increase among business executives who are not in the market for new or better jobs or promotions, who are well established and secure in their positions and have no reason to fear younger competition but who simply don't want to look too obviously older than their colleagues.

There's also a sharp increase in the number of retired men seeking cosmetic surgery. And you'd be surprised how many of these men have it done only because their wives had it done first and their egos can't stand a wife who looks younger. That's their vanity showing.

Frequently, too, there is the older man who is so impressed with the way his wife looks *and feels* after her facelift that he decides to have one too. Among those who have made the medical trek to the Lintilhac Clinic in Tahiti are Mr. and Mrs. Robert F. Skelton of Santa Monica, California. Bob Skelton is a retired optometrist, his wife a retired teacher. Both happily invited me to have a look at their new faces during my research in Papeete. Mrs. Skelton's facelift had been done the previous year and her husband was so impressed with it that he decided, without any nudging from her, that he needed some nips and tucks on his own face.

I had never met them before; I could only compare their new faces with the old ones in personal snapshots they showed me. The difference was striking but more significant was their mental attitude. I talked to them again some months later in Santa Monica. They were still ebulliently happy with their lifts.

"I think it's definitely the upcoming thing for men," said

Bob Skelton. "Why should it be only for women? And there's no reason to hide it, to try to keep it a secret. I'm telling everyone I know about it. But you have to be realistic. A facelift doesn't change your actual age—I'm sure a lot of people wish it could but it can't. I doubt if anyone really likes the thought of growing old, if you stop to think about it, and the certain reality that faces us in the end. A facelift doesn't change reality but it sure makes you *feel* different. It's hard for me to realize my age."

With his youthful new face he doesn't see any point now in telling his age. I don't blame him. But he doesn't mind saying he's taking his grandchildren on a camping trip—and hearing people tell him he doesn't look old enough to be a grandfather.

Bob P., a friend of mine, is an exceptionally youthful-looking sixty-two, tall and dark, lithe and lean, attractive and happily married. His wife, fifty-four, has not had a facelift and doesn't need one. Most people would say neither does Bob. But one day recently he looked in the mirror and made an instant decision to have one. His reason reflects the male counterpart of the darling-I'm-dripping (or drooping) approach.

"I suddenly didn't like what I saw in the mirror," he said. "When you get older, the skin falls. You see it all the time in older people. Mine isn't too noticeable yet to other people but it is to me and it annoys me. I have a few folds of loose skin around my lower jaw that I have to pull up tight when I shave. I've nicked myself a few times. Finally, I just decided—this is ridiculous. I'm very young in spirit, I'm in good health, I think of myself as being very young, so what's wrong with having these wattles cut off? I don't want to look twenty, I don't like faces that are drastically changed, I just want to look somewhere closer to how old I feel. I think that if there's something about your face that annoys you when you look in the mirror, and there's something that can be done about it surgically, the time has come when you need a facelift.

"My decision was as simple as that. What I see in the mirror annoys me, I don't intend to let it continue to annoy me, I want to be happy with myself." He'll soon be checking in for his facelift.

At the other end of the pole, of course, are men who somehow remain youthful and happy with themselves without artificial rejuvenation. Maurice Chevalier, one of the great entertainers of all time, once told me his secret of perpetual youth. He was seventy-eight but still going strong. Age hadn't dimmed his jaunty step and smile, his *joie de vivre,* or his timeless, irresistible charm.

"When you reach sixty," he said, "you have to decide what you like best in life—whether it is to be an artist and make love to an audience, or drink and run after girls and live it up. You have no more the strength to do everything, so you have to choose. I had five or six sincere passions of love, and at sixty I knew I could not go on doing everything, and I thought about it very seriously and I concluded that my greatest happiness was to be liked and respected by people for my work."

How did he keep in shape for his work? "I live the life of a boxer," he replied. Had he taken any of Europe's famed rejuvenation treatments so popular with Hollywood celebrities? Indeed he had not and he confessed to being a little old-fashioned about trying to improve upon nature, or changing the status quo with artificial rejuvenators or de-aging devices and beautifiers.

He touched his hand to his silvery-white hair and said proudly, "It's my own. I believe in naturalness. I have good friends who do all these other things—the treatments and injections and wrinkle removing. But for myself or my family, I would not approve. I do not believe in changing what God intended and when my work is finished, I will go—just the way I am.

"Age is a delusion anyhow, and a person's wrinkles can be

very attractive. It all depends on what's inside, or the look in a person's eyes.

"For myself I can say I am only myself—I am an old man. But I am a fresh old man. My terrific happiness is to be such an attraction at seventy-eight. This is the greatest gift that God has given me."

A New York critic once wrote, "Chevalier is a child with white hair. . . ."

But he had his own postscript for this. "Within you there must be enthusiasm and freshness," he said. "It's not a trick to learn. Either you have it, or you don't have it."

I'm sure this will be discouraging to the have-nots. But for those who, like Chevalier, do not believe in changing what God intended—and there are still many who don't—there is always the Lin Yutang solution that all old people, if they can, should go and live in China where age rather than youth is revered and where even a beggar with a white beard is treated with extra kindness.

But that's a long way to go just for the joy of growing old gracefully and with TLC.

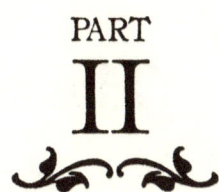

THE
FACE PEELERS:
Update

8

The Maschek Story:

Now It Can Be Told

The newest wrinkle in the Great Wrinkle Rip-off is the chemical face peel. The medical term is chemosurgery.

It is also called the "non-surgical" facelift and is done by swabbing the skin with a strong acid solution, giving you something like a second-degree burn and eventually a new face with skin as pink and fresh as a newborn baby's bottom.

Chemosurgery is not a new discovery; what is new is the increasing number of plastic surgeons now using it as an adjunct to their surgical facelifts and trying to perpetuate the myth that they're the only ones who know how to do it.

Only a few years back they were calling it quackery. In their opinion it's still quackery when done by lay operators, but okay if done by licensed MDs. They'll tell you it's "too delicate and hazardous" to be performed by "non-medical personnel" with "secret" formulas. The complication rate is purported to be "extremely low" when plastic surgeons do the treatment, but the perils of face peeling are "infinitely increased" if the work is done by a layman. In fact, you're apt to be scarred for life, they claim.

Typical of the warnings from organized medicine is this one by a medical science writer:

"The 'nonsurgical procedures' that promise to restore a sagging face are a waste of time and money, as anyone who has ever been seduced by their advertisements with their pie-in-the-sky promises will admit. The only way baggy skins can be made to fit the faces and necks once again is by a surgical procedure called a face lift performed by a highly trained plastic surgeon."

Personally, I've seen a thousand times more and bigger advertisements with pie-in-the-sky promises from plastic surgeons—usually with before-and-after pictures—than from "nonsurgical" operators but that may be only because I read the Los Angeles *Times*.

Also I am aware—and *you* should be too—that a chemical peel can't do as much for heavy jowling as a surgical facelift. Nor do the reputable practitioners of the chemical face peel, or "facial rejuvenation" as it is generally known, make any such claims. Their specialty is wrinkle removing, not jowl lifting. And at this they are as good as the plastic surgeons, sometimes better.

To say that the "nonsurgical procedures"—chemical face-lifts—are a waste of time and money unless performed by plastic surgeons is not only a gross misrepresentation of facts but a devious ploy in the whole facelift enchilada of cutthroat scalpel mongers with MD labels.

Moreover, such holier-than-peel pronouncements only compound the confusion of those who are trying to decide whether to have a surgical or chemical facelift, or both.

What it boils down to is whether you prefer the peel to the knife, and for the benefit of those still in limbo I think it's time to set the record straight.

Again, let me remind you that this book is not intended to be an endorsement of any one technique over another, nor of any facelifter, surgical or non-surgical. It is a guide to help *you* to decide whether you're *sure* you want a facelift, and if so where to go to get the best results that will please *you*.

Up to this chapter I still haven't had my face lifted but I'm still seriously thinking about it. When and if I do, you may be sure that I'll choose a lifter whom I have thoroughly investigated.

In the field of facial rejuvenation, I doubt if anyone has ever been more thoroughly investigated and medically guillotined than Miriam Maschek, a petite, blond, non-medical practitioner in Miami, whose fantastic results at wrinkle removing stirred up a national controversy, captured the imagination of millions, and undoubtedly added many a wrinkle to the furrowed brows of AMA bloodhounds, who for years doggedly tried to put her out of business.

And for a while I doggedly tried to help them.

As a reporter for the Chicago *Tribune,* I had earned some recognition (and a few prizes) for exposing medical quacks, usually with the help of the AMA's Bureau of Investigation, the FDA, and state licensing agencies. As an assignment for the *Tribune,* and in co-operation with the AMA, I went to Miami well armed and backgrounded to expose Miriam Maschek as a fraud. I can smell a quack a mile away. Miriam Maschek wasn't one of them. After months of checking her out, I returned to Miami and spent three weeks following the day-by-day, step-by-step chemical rejuvenation of a forty-year-old woman, Anne White, and wrote a fourteen-part series on the peeling process, which was syndicated in many papers.

In one of the articles, I wrote: "Neither The Tribune nor the medical profession recommends 'facial rejuvenation' treatments. As a reporter, I can merely say that in many years of investigating medical claims in all categories, I have never met a person who worked with greater care, patience, and artistry —as well as real concern for her client—than this woman." (Miriam Maschek)

That was written in February 1960. My statement still stands. Miriam has since died but her technique of facial rejuvenation through chemical peeling is still being carried on by her non-medical husband, Francis, in collaboration with an MD, a licensed, Board certified dermatologist.

Because the Maschek Treatment has become so famous and controversial, I feel it warrants an updated reprise for readers of this book. Thousands of men and women have had the treatment; thousands more are wondering about it.

In the twenty years since I first set out to expose the Mascheks as quacks, I have returned to Miami many times, observed scores of their patients in various stages of the chemical peeling process, interviewed hundreds who have been happily peeled with results as remarkable and lasting as plastic surgery, often more so.

Paradoxically, the plastic surgeons now resorting to peels are using basically the same chemical formula used by the Mascheks.

Of course they'll scream to high heaven when they read this and they'll deny it. And probably most of them don't even know they're using the Maschek formula. But the plastic surgeons in Miami know it and some will even admit it—off the record.

In fact two of Miami's leading plastic surgeons as well as two top dermatologists told me, "Face peeling is more a cosmetic procedure. We're not as well qualified to do it as the lay operators here." When I asked specifically if they meant the Mascheks, they said yes. A couple of them volunteered that they couldn't be bothered with doing peels because the technique of doing them properly was too "complicated" and time-consuming. "When I get a patient who wants or needs a peel along with a facelift, I send them to the Mascheks," one said. Another of the plastic surgeons frankly admitted confidentially, "Of course, we're not supposed to say this but anything the plastic surgeons know about face peeling they've learned from lay operators."

I first heard about Miriam Maschek from a Chicago business executive who called me and said, "I've got a helluva story for you. How would you like to turn back the clock and look twenty years younger?" Ho ho, I thought, that would be a helluva story but not the kind he was thinking about. His wife,

as I had suspected, had just had her face done, and he was ecstatic over the results.

It was this call that led to my assignment in Miami, the investigation of the Mascheks and their treatment, and the subsequent series on Anne White.

Mrs. White, wife of a Miami businessman, mother of
three, was an attractive woman, athletic, and with a trim, lithe
figure. Her only problem was her face. Though only forty, her
face was wrinkled and leathery and spattered with brown
spots. Doctors had told her she was born with an "old" skin.

"I wouldn't mind looking forty if only my skin didn't look
sixty," she said.

A dermatologist had removed some fifty of her small
brown spots, caused by the sun and sometimes called surface
skin cancers, over the previous ten years but they kept coming
back. She was a sun worshipper and admitted it; she lived in
the sun, swam in it, fished, golfed, and water-skied in it—and
tried to hide what it did to her under a heavy mask of pancake
makeup. When the makeup was removed, she had dried-up,
weather-beaten skin.

Her dermatologist gave his approval for her to be treated
by Miriam Maschek. I then accompanied Mrs. White to the
doctor's office for her physical examination, required of all
Maschek clients. She passed it easily. The doctor wrote pre-
scriptions for several kinds of pills—mostly sedatives and tran-
quilizers. He told me, "Ethically I cannot recommend this"
(the Maschek treatment) "because the medical profession
doesn't approve of it. But I'd trust my own wife to Mrs.
Maschek when she's ready to have her face done."

Mrs. Maschek, then fifty-three but with a freshly rejuvenated fortyish face, was a rather shy, serious, blue-and-wide-
eyed Pennsylvania Dutch woman whose ambition was to be a
nurse and who seemed to be doing a pretty good job of it after
stumbling accidentally into the fountain-of-youth business. A
Frenchwoman named Antoinette la Gasse, famous on the West
Coast in the thirties and early forties for rejuvenating movie
stars, had employed Miriam as her assistant, then willed her

the so-called "secret" formula, which dozens of others claim was willed to them.

"There's nothing secret or mysterious about it. You just have to know how to do it," Mrs. Maschek explained, as she started in on the rejuvenation of Anne White, permitting me to be an eyewitness to the non-surgical, non-medical miracle of de-aging Anne's "old" skin.

"I don't know what you call my formula," Miriam said. "It isn't facial rejuvenation. That's what quacks do. I'm not medical. I don't have a degree. I'm not a beautician. I didn't go to beauty school. The beauticians say I have to go to a beauty school. I wouldn't mind, but I do faces—not heads."

Actually, the Mascheks were licensed as "facial rejuvenators." The state of Florida permits "facial rejuvenation," and the Mascheks were operating quite openly under a state license obtained in 1957 by their attorney, Robert Riddle.

Their so-called "secret" formula was—and still is—composed of chemical compounds well known in the medical profession. It had been investigated and approved by the FDA. In December 1958, the then State Drug Inspector, Walter G. Stelts, reported, "Since our decision as to its [the solution's] use by Mrs. Maschek at the present time is favorable, she in no way would be in violation of the Florida Pure Food, Drug and Cosmetic act by the use of same." He added that Mrs. Maschek's "fine reputation, her knowledge of the work, her character and ability were important factors in rendering the decision"

Before retiring for the night, Anne White was given two tablets—one a mild pain reliever, the other a tranquilizer—which had been prescribed by the examining physician.

The next morning she had her last chewable food—a breakfast of warm Danish rolls, freshly squeezed orange juice, coffee, and a vitamin pill. At 11 A.M. she was given another pill, also prescribed by the doctor. Then she telephoned her husband to cheer him up, while Miriam Maschek and her husband, Francis—they worked as a team—prepared the tapes, the hot water bottles, the ether, and swab sticks.

At noon they went to work on Mrs. White, cleaning her

face first with ether, then applying their bottle formula with careful strokes of cotton-wrapped swab sticks. Immediately after this application, hundreds of tiny, odd-shaped strips of adhesive tape were slowly and carefully taped over the forehead and nose, one over the other in strange patterns, until they lay in heaped mounds.

The two things of utmost importance in their process, the Mascheks explained, were the timing and taping. The mounds of curiously shaped tapes stayed on for X number of hours—or days—and this was timed to the minute. The Mascheks kept written records, practically hour by hour, on each client.

As soon as the tapes came off—clean and with no loose skin peels—the exposed surface was then covered with a brown powder containing an iodine compound, which hardened into a mask.

The neck and face were treated section by section, the forehead and nose first, then the left side (always more difficult to treat than the right, they explained), the right side, and finally the neck.

After watching the entire process for three weeks, I knew what Inspector Stelts meant when he told me, "It's not so much what they use but how they use it."

I also knew why it was too complicated and time-consuming for plastic surgeons to bother with, or anyone else, for that matter, except someone totally dedicated; and why it could be dangerous in the hands of people dedicated more to dollars than de-wrinkling craftsmanship, whether they were lay operators or MDs with the AMA's Gold Seal of Approval.

In the first hours after taping, clients usually experience a stinging or burning sensation, in varying degrees. Anne White was up and prancing around immediately after her first treatment—on the forehead and nose. But after treatment No. 2—the left cheek—she wrote to me on a slate, which was provided for her because she was not permitted to talk, "It's hot as hell!"

Her mouth was taped. Her right cheek and eye were swollen—almost shut. She peeked at herself in a hand mirror, then wrote: "My husband called and wanted to come and see me this afternoon. I'm glad I said no. I would really scare him."

She looked like a zombie.

"Is it as bad as going to a dentist?" I asked.

"No," she wrote. "It's just a stinging, pulsating sensation. But it isn't unbearable. I wouldn't care if it burned all night, I'm so enthused about it."

"Have you ever been sorry—or scared—even for one second that you started this?"

She shook her head so hard at first that I thought she might crack her mask, then calmed down and wrote, "It looks worse than it really is."

"What do you miss most?"

"Brushing my teeth and a good shower." Then she added: "P.S. The heat is tapering off."

Francis Maschek brought her a tall glass of beef stew whipped up in a blender. Anne drank her supper, bypassed dessert, and took a glass of black coffee, which she sipped through a plastic tube. Then she wrote, "P.S. The burning has gone."

She still had two more treatments to go, and then ten days of the hard, tight feeling of wrinkled-skin years vanishing behind her zombie mask.

At the end of three weeks her face looked as though she'd had a rather bright pink sunburn. "It feels a little tight—just like a sunburn," she said. "But I've had much worse burns at home, frying chicken."

Anne White's new face bore little resemblance to her old one. All her lines, wrinkles, and brown spots were gone. She had rose-petal skin and big blue eyes like saucers. Even the droopy skin on her eyelids had gone—don't ask me where.

A week later she looked better; the redness and swelling had diminished. But what about a year later? Five years? Ten years? Now?

One of the first questions most people ask is, How long does a facelift last? The answer generally is eight to ten years, depending on how well you take care of it.

I did a follow-up report on Anne White a year after her "facial rejuvenation," and another five years later, in February 1966. At forty-six she looked much younger and more attractive than she had at forty with her prematurely aged skin. Under bright lights, I poked and scrutinized for wrinkles or brown spots with no luck.

I have seen her several times since then during assignments in Miami, and most recently while I was there interviewing MDs for this book.

The last time I saw her Anne White was still alive and well and wrinkleless despite the dire predictions of the medical fraternity regarding the chemical face peel in the hands of non-medical personnel. In the twenty years since her peel she'd never had keloids, kidney problems, scars, or any of those other perils-of-peeling attributed exclusively to lay operators.

Her face has stood up amazingly well in the chronological age grist mill. At sixty she looked better than she did at forty, though she admitted that she had taken much better care of her skin since her peel. She was still swimming and playing golf but always made sure her face was well protected with a sunscreen and/or a hat. She was also considering a return trip to the Maschek clinic for a touch-up peel. "I'm not bad for sixty, don't you think? But my face has given me a new lease on life for twenty years now," she said, "and I intend to renew the lease while I'm ahead."

9

Old Hat with New Ribbons

I have purposely avoided going into the technical details and terminology of the various types of cosmetic surgery. That is best done by plastic surgeons and there are plenty of books on the market as well as scientific papers and journals in medical libraries for anyone who wants to wade through them.

I doubt if many people who have open-heart surgery or a cholecystectomy, for example, are all that interested in how it's done. When they have a doctor they trust, they put themselves in his hands and hope for the best.

I am assuming that most of you reading this book feel the same way. In the area of facelifting, however, it is becoming increasingly difficult to find a doctor you trust, not only because so many MDs have hopped on the cosmetic roller coaster but because it's open sesame for unscrupulous operators and outright charlatans.

This is especially true in the area of non-surgical lifts, chemosurgery, "facial rejuvenation," or chemical face peeling —whatever you choose to call it.

In spite of my personal investigation and conclusions on

the Maschek method over a span of twenty years, I must say unequivocally that the chemical face peel in the wrong hands can be extremely dangerous if not disastrous.

The reason is technical but I'll try to simplify it as much as possible because it's something that every reader of this book should understand.

The basic ingredient of chemosurgery is phenol acid or trichloroacetic acid.

The deep face peel is sometimes called the "phenol peel."

Phenol, in layman's language, is carbolic acid.

Now, don't let this scare you away from a face peel if that's what you want. Just make doubly sure you find a peeler who knows for sure what he's doing.

"Phenol Chemosurgery" for removal of facial wrinkles is now a commonly accepted procedure as an adjunct to the surgical facelift, as evidenced in an abundance of medical literature on the subject and by the growing number of plastic surgeons who use it, whether they know how or not.

But the real problem is the ease with which anyone can lay hands on the basic chemical formula and set up shop as a "facial rejuvenator."

Finding a qualified practitioner of chemosurgery is far more difficult than finding a qualified plastic surgeon.

It is not likely that a layman with no medical training at all will just go out and buy a scalpel and hang out his shingle as a plastic surgeon. But in the face-peeling business anyone can do it. The actual chemistry of the peel, available in medical literature, is easily grasped by any intelligent laymen, and some not so intelligent who add a little more or less of this or that to make the solution mild, medium, or strong for a light, medium, or deep peel. Or whatever.

How would you like to have your face dabbed with carbolic acid by an abortionist? You get the general idea.

During my investigation of the Mascheks and their treatment I was told by Inspector Stelts, "I've watched them work. And I've seen their clients—both before and after. There's no question that they know what they're doing. There's never been a complaint against them, except from beauticians." (Because they were operating without a beauticians' license.)

But, Stelts emphasized: *"The biggest danger to the public in such a treatment is in fly-by-night quack competitors trying to imitate it."*

For this reason, he said, he gave his "favorable" decision on the Mascheks *only on condition that they would not market their product, or train others to use it, or publicly disclose their formula or technique.*

The Mascheks were adhering strictly to these conditions and I respected their request not to reveal their formula or the *proportions*—which are important. Thus started the "secret formula" brouhaha.

Ironically, it was an MD on the AMA's own Cosmetics Committee who was responsible for bringing the much touted "secret formula" to public attention, thus opening the door for the fly-by-night quacks.

So incensed were the Hippocratic High Priests at my stories on the Mascheks that they released what they assumed to be their "secret formula" to a reporter on a competition newspaper who promptly popped down to Miami and did his own exposé on the Mascheks by interviewing the MDs who think that only MDs should do face peels. And they're not too hard to find.

The real coup, in the AMA's Hippocratical eyes, was an admission from the Mascheks that they used a phenol base in their formula.

They did not disclose their exact formula and never have. It wasn't necessary, with the AMA leaping into the fray.

The upshot of all the uproar, with a deep-peel formula now published and up for grabs, was a proliferation of weirdos just waiting to cash in on a good thing.

And they were not all lay operators.

Soon after my Maschek series ran its course, a bona fide, certified, well-connected New York City dermatologist (MD) opened a "rejuvenation" salon in Connecticut with skin-peel techniques which he claimed were the "latest advances in medical science." They were loosely—very loosely—patterned after the Maschek treatment. The doctor's chief technician was a licensed cosmetician formerly with a swank hairdressing salon in New York.

"We specialize in wrinkles, scars, and sagging skin," she told me. "We do only faces. And sometimes necks down to the collar bone. No shoulders or hands."

The doctor's medical associate was another dermatologist (MD) operating in Daytona Beach, Florida, doing chemical facelifts in his office. Patients stayed in nearby motels. I took one look at the setup—and ran!

My subsequent investigation found the two MDs to be using the phenol-base formula without the taping masks which are generally acknowledged to be crucial to the degree of success achieved in chemosurgery.

"Some we put in tapes and bandages, some we don't. It's a highly individualized thing," the technician told me.

Patients were fed liquid diets through a plastic straw, à la the Mascheks, with one notable difference. In the Connecticut rejuvenation salon, a remodeled farmhouse operating under a cosmetician's license, the physical discomforts of de-aging were eased with eggnogs in a variety of flavors—brandy, Bourbon, scotch, rum, vodka, and so on.

A Chicago working woman who had saved her money for a trip east to be rejuvenated reported: "It was a nightmare. The house reminded me of an Alfred Hitchcock murder movie. Everyone was loaded—on eggnogs. They were going to charge me $1,500 for a new face and no neck. I should get a new face without the neck?"

She walked out and took the next plane to Miami.

I talked with the financial backers of this particular Connecticut-Florida MD wrinkle-removing team. The principal backers were a former insurance salesman and his wife, who told me quite frankly that they just went into wrinkle removing because they got tired of the insurance business. They planned to open rejuvenation salons in Texas and California along with the one in Connecticut.

"People are extremely puzzled about how to define us," they said "There is no decent middle ground between the beauty parlor and the medical profession. We think we're a cosmetic treatment, not medical.

"Our treatment needs no doctor for the application. This is done by non-medical technicians. But we always have one doctor on call."

They said "several other doctors" besides the New York dermatologist "work closely with us" but they could not reveal their names. "They prefer it this way."

I was unable to locate the dermatologist at either his Connecticut salon or his Daytona Beach, Florida, office. I was told he hadn't been around much since the story of his new rejuvenation treatment was published in a national weekly magazine.

A check with the dermatology department of a New York medical center with which he was affiliated revealed that he had been inactive for several years prior to his retirement two years before his alleged skin-peel discoveries. A spokesman for the medical center said skin-peeling experiments had been tried many years ago and then discontinued "for many reasons."

"Our attitude is quite the same," he added. "This is old hat with new ribbons. Anything Dr. X is doing is completely on his own and independent of us. But it's not the sort of thing that would get by the chairman of the department if he were still with us."

Meanwhile I learned that a Chicago MD who was a well-known abortionist was planning to install a rejuvenating "technician" in his office. He would have his own "secret formula" similar to Dr. X's, who incidentally was soon out of business, but the fly-by-nights began mushrooming and the Mascheks were soon swamped with repair jobs on faces botched up by their imitators.

Where and how did "chemosurgery"—the chemical face peel—originate?

Its tangled ancestry is not only intriguingly bizarre but quite relevant to the sole purpose of this book—to help readers decide whether they want a facelift and if so, what kind and by whom.

Superficial skin peeling has been traced back to the early Egyptians, who made an abrasive paste consisting of alabaster particles in milk and honey. Chemosurgery is comparatively new in the medical arsenal. Phenol (carbolic acid) was a popular disinfectant at the close of the nineteenth century, and in the 1920s and 1930s was used to remove birthmarks. Doctors were aware of the gamut of chemicals now used by facial rejuvenators but in the early years they found the peel less reliable than skin planing, or dermabrasion.

Most of today's deep-peel facelifts, with their phenol-base formula, taping and powdering techniques, are derived directly or indirectly from the famous lay operator, Antoinette la Gasse, a mysterious and legendary Frenchwoman who, as mentioned earlier, was known for clandestinely rejuvenating the jaded faces of movie stars during Hollywood's Golden Era, the thirties and forties.

The story goes that Antoinette's father was a French physician who was treating soldiers after World War I for powder burns of the face with phenol solutions, a not uncommon treatment at that time. His nurse, on one occasion, in a fortuitous bit of improvisation, covered the unattractive treated areas with adhesive tape.

The doctor noticed the cosmetic improvement of the patient's skin, and went on to refine the formula and technique in his practice. Antoinette, who had worked as a nurse in her father's office, immigrated to the United States, bringing with her the formula and technique.

She was an immediate hit in Hollywood. Naturally, she had her skirmishes with the medical profession. She was once arrested and charged with unauthorized medical practice, but the charges were later dropped. She remained in business and her business thrived. By the late 1940s, she had taken on two apprentices who were to become even more famous—or infamous in the files of the AMA. They were Cora Galenti and Miriam Maschek.

The sordid and sad saga of Cora Galenti has been thoroughly researched and documented by former *Newsweek* correspondent Patrick M. McGrady, Jr., in his book *The Youth Doctors*. Cora was put out of business for reasons, he concludes, that "had little if anything to do with her skill or lack of skill as a youth doctor."

Both Cora and Miriam claimed that the beloved Antoinette had "willed" her rejuvenation formula to them when she died of cancer in 1952 or thereabouts.

Probably unmentioned in the legacy was Antoinette's lover, Monsieur Adelaide Giroux, who became husband number two for Cora Galenti, and the Mascheks figured that had something to do with Cora's usurpation of Antoinette's fountain-of-youth formula. According to Cora, Mrs. Maschek stole the formula.

Anyhow the two rejuvenators went their separate ways, Miriam to Miami and Cora to Nevada when she was hounded out of California by medical authorities.

As Patrick McGrady points out, "Both Cora Galenti and Miriam Maschek were getting fantastic results, by and large."

As accurately as I can interpret it, both Cora and Miriam, during their apprenticeship with Antoinette, probably learned enough about her formula and technique to carry on her work with some creative skill; obviously they did or they couldn't have continued to work on so many celebrity clients over the years; word travels fast in these circles—one mistake and you're out, Buster!

However, their come-on approach was quite different and Miss Galenti eventually did herself in, not for practicing medicine without a license (for which she was twice arrested) but for mail fraud. She boldly and blatantly advertised in the women's pages and magazines:

"To ALL Women . . . who wish to recapture Youthful Loveliness! Take 20–30 years from your face and neck. Internationally famous beauty consultant offers new faces for old without surgery! There is no cutting, no burning, no peeling, no pain, and very little discomfort in the Galenti process of facial rejuvenation that completely erases 20, 30, and sometimes 40 years of sags and wrinkles. The secret is Cora Galenti's secret . . . a precious formula that has been in her family for more than 150 years. The process is simplicity itself!"

I'm not sure how the precious formula that has been in her family for more than 150 years squares with her claim that her formula was willed to her by Antoinette, but in any case U.S. postal inspectors went after her for the obvious falsehoods contained in her ads ("no burning, no peeling, no pain . . .") and she was tried for mail fraud and convicted. She is reported to be still discreetly plying her trade in Tijuana, Mexico.

Meanwhile, the Mascheks survived their own hassles with the medical czars in fine shape.

In denigrating their lay competitors, the MDs inadvertently triggered a flurry of independent research into the phenol face peeling, often with results most embarrassing to the Establishment.

The Mascheks were invited to work as consultants in the (skin) cancer research department at the University of Rochester in New York. They demonstrated their method to head dermatologists. Soon after this two of Miami's leading dermatologists paid a visit to Rochester, then began exploring peels together at the University of Miami and writing papers on their findings.

At the Southern California School of Medicine, a professor of dermatology found that "phenol application [shows results] . . . in some cases superior to those from surgical planing [dermabrasion]."

And a prominent Los Angeles plastic surgeon and his wife conducted their own phenol tests and found that the peel was not only a useful tool, but far superior in some respects to anything accomplished by dermabrasion or plastic surgery.

He later patented his own formula and published it in medical journals, claiming, however, that it was too dangerous to be used by lay operators—despite the fact that it strongly resembled the one used by Cora Galenti and Miriam Maschek. The MD also made a special point of warning the public against charlatans. By way of illustration he emphasized that there had been a "phenol death" in Los Angeles during a "face peel" by a lay operator.

After extensive investigation into the Galenti saga, including the M.D.'s allegation of a "phenol death," author Patrick McGrady had this to say on the subject:

"Dr. ———— erred in accusing a lay operator of causing a 'phenol death.' The Los Angeles death he likely was referring to later was determined to have been caused by heart attack. I have been unable to trace *any* death to the facial application of phenol by a lay operator. There have, on the other hand, been recorded instances of phenol-induced deaths by MDs trying to remove baby blemishes and scarification."

I have been soundly chastised in the medical journals for "extolling the work of lay operators," and I will be again when the MDs read these chapters. I'm sure writer McGrady was too. But I doubt if the whole kit and kaboodle of Hippocratic MDs—shouldn't that be spelled Hypocritic?—have spent a tenth as much time and effort checking out the lay operators as we have.

I believe, with Mr. McGrady, that most people would prefer to be treated by qualified plastic surgeons. I agree with him that it seems the summit of hypocrisy for the MDs to feign shock or outrage when patients seek out lay operators for face peels. If the phenol face peel properly belongs only to qualified MDs, then why haven't more qualified MDs taken the trouble to learn how to do it?

Furthermore, in fairness to all the readers of this book, I cannot conscientiously omit an important fact that somewhat parallels Mr. McGrady's experience and will send MDs into a tizzy.

I, too, have been unable to trace *any* death to the facial application of phenol by a lay operator; nor for that matter any serious injuries or scars, though I've read about them in the medical literature.

There are, on the other hand, at this very moment, two patients in the Maschek clinic in Miami who are there because of botched-up jobs by plastic surgeons. In one case the MD snipped too much skin off her eyelids. The other is a patient undergoing chemical repairs for scars on a badly hacked-up nose. The doctor's knife slipped during her nose job and ran through her nose.

Well . . . nobody's perfect.

10

Ghost Peeler for MDs

Miriam Maschek's husband, Francis, had always worked closely with her. They were a devoted couple, deeply religious, and totally dedicated to their work. They were beloved by everyone who knew them.

They ran an efficient, well-ordered, impeccably immaculate, and beautifully appointed establishment, which they called the House of Renaissance, or sometimes, jokingly, the "wrinkle farm."

On several occasions I stayed with them, when there was a room available. No, I already told you, I did not have my face done. But I had the opportunity and rare privilege of an inside look at everything that went on in the place, from the phenol face peels—and hands and arms, too—to the twenty-four-hour TLC and pampering of patients, including the marvelous concoctions Francis whipped up in his blender for them to sip for their supper or midnight or mid-morning snacks. If anyone wanted fresh blended watermelon at 3 A.M., *voilà*, there it was, with the plastic straw to drink it.

The thing that impressed me most, next to the wrinkle-free

faces that came out of the zombie tape masks, was the pervading aura of happiness and uplift that went along with the facelift. The Mascheks provided their clients with positive-thinking books to read and Miriam always smilingly admonished them to: "Think happy thoughts or your wrinkles will come back."

Her own happy thoughts turned to heartache in later years. Miriam was a frail woman, and Francis waited on her hand and foot, serving her breakfast and dinner in bed, doing everything he could to spare her strength and hands for her work. She had the hands of an artist. The placement of the tiny tapes to form the facial mask requires great digital dexterity and sensitivity. And good eyesight. When a long bout with pneumonia left Miriam with an eye infection, she began turning over more and more of the taping and peeling work to Francis. Her hands were still steady but her spirit was broken as encroaching blindness set in. Clients who still flocked to their glamorous "wrinkle farm" were willing to entrust their faces to Francis. With Miriam's help he had developed his own digital dexterity and sensitivity and had been doing all the faces—with no complaints—for two years before Miriam's death in 1970 (from pneumonia and complicated respiratory problems, but probably as much from a broken heart as anything else).

I was down on the "wrinkle farm" again during this difficult transition in the Maschek Treatment. I was probably one of the last to talk to Miriam Maschek before she died and one of the first to be given *carte blanche* inspection of their present clinical techniques for comparative purposes in researching this book.

Francis Maschek has continued to carry on the work as a licensed facial rejuvenator in collaboration with Dr. B. G. Gross, a licensed and Board certified dermatologist, and former instructor in the Department of Dermatology at the University of Miami School of Medicine.

There is no doubt that this new affiliation with a bona fide

MD has taken some of the onus off the Maschek peel and elevated it to a sufficient level of respectability to be acceptable to the plastic surgeons who now send the clinic patients for face peels.

With publication of their own scientific paper, "Phenol Chemosurgery for Removal of Deep Facial Wrinkles," in medical journals, it now appears that Gross and Maschek are the new Deans of the Deep Peel, using basically the same formula which beleaguered lay operators have been using for more than half a century—ever since the fabled Frenchwoman "Antoinette," as Hollywood knew her, began rejuvenating the jaded movie stars.

"Is it still Antoinette's formula?" I asked Francis recently.

"It's still the same," he said. "And there has never been any secret about it. But you have to know how to use it. It's the techniques of applying the solution and the tape masks that make it different and unique. I've given the formula to topnotch plastic surgeons but they don't know how to use it, they can't take the time to learn the techniques. It isn't taught in medical schools and it isn't something you can learn to do just from reading the technical papers. That's doing it by trial and error.

"It's a difficult and delicate procedure, and it can be dangerous if it isn't done properly throughout all the various stages. To learn it requires time and patience and personal observation and practice. You have to be personally taught and trained."

Francis personally trained Dr. Gross in the non-surgical operation.

"I've offered to teach other medical men but they don't want to be taught by a lay operator. I wouldn't teach it to another lay person though," he said, "because I wouldn't want to be responsible for creating a monster. I'd be taking too big a chance. There are a lot of people who would love to know how to do it, but all they're thinking about is the money, not the patients. And this is serious business, when you're working with faces. If something goes wrong on the body, you can cover up the scars, but not on the face. You can't fool around with phenol. You can't just teach anybody who comes in off the street."

While most MDs in my research have been disappointingly coy about revealing their own peel formulas and techniques, or in giving credit to anyone but themselves, Dr. Gross discussed his conversion from orthodox medical techniques to the Maschek method with surprising candor.

"Practically every plastic surgeon and dermatologist has dabbled in it" (face peeling) "with very spotty and irregular results," he said. "It was not until I came here and watched Francis that I began to understand why our techniques were inadequate. I was astounded at his technique. It was so much more aggressive than anything I would have dared to do in my practice. I've brought many of my doctor friends here and they're astounded, too, when they see why their peels are not as successful as Francis's."

Dr. Gross had been in private practice as a dermatologist for eleven years; he gave up his practice to become an apprentice in the Maschek techniques of facial rejuvenation.

"I was quite aware of what I was doing," he told me. "I knew I'd be jeered by my medical colleagues. I've lived in this area a long time so I'd heard plenty about the Mascheks. I knew they were frowned on by the AMA. But I knew from my own patients that they were turning out good work—better than anything I could do.

"With the growing demand for facelifts, I think there's a crying need for qualified MDs, especially plastic surgeons and dermatologists, to learn how to do peels with safe and effective results. If we can learn something from an experienced and trained lay operator like Francis Maschek, I think it's to our advantage as well as the public's.

"His ethical standards are as high as any in the medical profession, higher than those of some MDs. He works with more careful precision than any doctor I know. He has shown his techniques to the physicians who have attempted to crucify him, and even 'ghosted' face peels for some of them.

"Everything they know about peels they have learned either directly or indirectly from him."

Francis admitted that he had been a reluctant "ghost peeler" for some MDs who didn't know how to do peels—but didn't want to admit it to their patients. He no longer "ghosts" for them; if they want their patients peeled, they can send them to him.

He doesn't want to take any chance of being shafted for the laying on of hands in an MD's domain, even though his services were solicited. Actually, the practice of "ghosting" is not uncommon in cosmetic surgery; one doctor does one side of the face and another doctor does the other side, without telling the patient.

What makes the Gross-Maschek technique different from those readily available in textbooks of cosmetic surgery? Capsuled in lay terms:

1. Application of the phenol solution is done by special bulky cotton swab sticks, not the ordinary Q-tips used by most doctors. The solution can't be controlled or applied evenly with Q-tips, they say. Francis makes the swab sticks himself— out of chopsticks! The squared ends of the chopsticks are flattened and wrapped with a one-and-a-half- to two-inch-wide strip of cotton, which acts as a reservoir and eliminates streaking.

2. Swabbing is continued until a *gray* cast appears on the skin, not white, which is where most peelers stop.

3. The most important key to the success of the peel is the use and application of the *tape mask*. This is also the most complicated and difficult part of the process to learn. The adhesive tapes are cut into several different lengths, widths, and shapes to conform to the contours of the face and applied in several layers, left on for varying lengths of time, removed and followed by a powdering and creaming technique, and etcetera.

And that's as much as you need to know about it.

I don't want to be responsible for some screwball going out and buying chopsticks and adhesive tape and messing around with anyone's face.

But this is enough to give you a general idea of why more qualified MDs don't go in for phenol peels and why those who do may get only a few superficial wrinkles removed.

There are a few modifications and innovations in the non-surgical facelift process as it is performed today by Dr. Gross and Francis Maschek.

They now do the whole face and neck at one time rather than in sections. This has cut down the total treatment time from three weeks to twelve days. They have refined the technique to virtually eliminate any line of demarcation where the chemical treatment has ended. The demarcation line in a deep face peel has always been a significant cosmetic problem for darker-skinned patients. But they have treated a large number of Spanish and South American patients, some with very dark skin, with surprisingly good results.

With the installation of Dr. Gross, the name of the Maschek rejuvenation emporium was changed, in deference to his MD specialty, to the Derma-Lift Salon.

He defends the face*lift* connotation, long considered the special prerogative of plastic surgeons.

"The word *facelift* is a misnomer in plastic surgery," he says. "What it really is, is a neck-lift, taking all that turkey wattle and tucking it up behind the ears. It does nothing above the chin."

A properly performed chemical peel, he explained, is more than a mere peel. It tightens and lifts not only the neck but the whole face from the chin up.

"What we're doing is a real facelift," he said.

And he's so sold on it that he has completely abandoned

the old orthodox standby of his medical specialty, dermabrasion, or skin planing.

The Derma-Lift Salon is equipped with all the latest, up-
to-date medical precautionary machines, including a heart
monitor. In my investigation, I have seen few if any private
clinics for facelifting better equipped or staffed. (There are almost as many in-help as patients.)

Francis Maschek has remarried and his new wife is a
glamorous touch-up to the Derma-Lift operation. Her name
may be familiar. She is Jacqueline Stallone, mother of "Sly"
(Sylvester) or "Rocky" Stallone, the movie star with all that
macho. Jacqueline, an exotic cross-breed of Hedy Lamarr and
Rosalind Russell, is a beauty-and-youth expert in her own
right, and when you're finished with your "derma-lift," you get
a free beauty-clinic trip with her and explicit instructions on
how to manipulate your false eyelashes.

The price tag on the whole enchilada (excluding hands
and arms, at $250 per pair) is only $3,000—cheap compared
with the going rate in many nip-and-clip joints.

But before you hop the next plane to Miami, read on.

11

To Peel or Not to Peel . . .?

That Is the Question

Assuming you've decided to have a facelift and are torn between the choice of having it done surgically or non-surgically, the question boils down to:

Do you want it done with the knife or the burn?

The answer is mostly psychological.

It's a little like asking, Do you prefer to be cremated or buried?

Some people have a psychological hang-up, or phobia, about being burned, buried, drowned, knifed, asphyxiated, *ad infinitum*.

In facelifting, fortunately, the torturous decision-making—often more painful than the facelift—narrows down to only two alternatives, scalpel or phenol.

Your choice depends on what you fear most—a *slip of the knife* or *the depth of the burn*.

Personally, in my twenty-odd years of scrutinizing faces lifted by both scalpel and phenol, I have never seen any gross disfigurements from either of them (though, believe me, I've searched!), nor any evidence that the one technique is superior to the other, technically or aesthetically. It all depends on what you want in a facelift.

Some crazies want to look twenty again when they're fifty, and there are plenty of MD crazies who are willing to oblige. Just bring in that long-gone-bloom-of-youth snapshot. You can get a cut or peel job that will roll off as many years as you want. Almost.

But if you opt for the peel, there are certain things you should know:

• It changes your skin *texture,* which plastic surgery does not.

• You have a newborn baby-pink skin which the surgeon's scalpel can't give you—*BUT . . .*

• You can't go out in the sun again for at least three months, preferably *NEVER.* Practically all doctors agree on this one point—avoid exposure to the sun. But with the chemical peel there are no ifs, ands, and buts—you stay out of the sun with your newborn baby skin.

Some people think it's worth the price, some don't.

In my interviews with hundreds of patients who have had chemical facelifts, I asked why they chose this method rather than the more conventional surgical facelifts. Their answers were about equally divided between:

[a] I didn't want an operation; I'm afraid of the knife.

[b] I've seen some of their faces (Mascheks') and that's good enough for me.

Personal recommendations are valuable in helping to choose between certain facelift techniques and doctors. But they must be weighed against a considerable bulwark of evidence, particularly in chemosurgery, that the phenol lift is not one to be recommended lightly.

Even the most highly qualified plastic surgeons admit they run a risk in performing the peel.

Medical experts warn that the peel, when done at the same time as a facelift, should be confined to small areas of the face, such as around the lips or forehead; *but an entire face peel must be performed separately, well after the face has recovered from the facelift operation.*

Yet, a top plastic surgeon in Palm Springs is turning out faces with total double-lifts, both surgical and full face peels, at one whack. A real whiz kid. So far he hasn't been around long enough to run a wrinkle poll on recidivism.

The face peel in the proper hands can give dramatic results. So can a surgical facelift. We have to settle for one or the other. It's a predatory and monopolistic ball of wax. Personally, if I'm going to entrust my face to a plastic surgeon, I'll choose the one who tells me frankly, "I don't do peels because I'm not qualified."

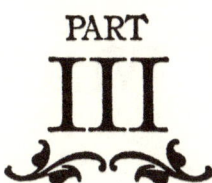

ROUNDUP
TIME

(Cosmetic Surgery)

12

What Are the Risks?

It depends on who is answering the question—the plastic surgeon, the dermatologist, the repairman, the patient, the beautician. Most doctors will tell you that beauticians are not qualified to pass judgment on facelifts. Be that as it may, they do anyway and women listen to them. Beauticians are usually the first to see a patient fresh from the scalpel or peel; generally they continue seeing her each week, unless she switches hairdressers; in many salons at least 50 per cent of the customers have had facelifts, and so beauty operators surely have a good basis for comparison. They see all the botched-up jobs and in a good many cases it's the beautician who tells his client where to go for her repair work.

Practically every plastic surgeon I have talked to has boastfully volunteered that *he* is the one who did the repair work on So-and-so's face. In Beverly Hills a top plastic surgeon, who specializes in eyes, claims that 50 per cent of his work is repairing botched-up eye jobs done by other surgeons.

Forty per cent of all patients who come to the Derma-Lift Salon in Miami have already had plastic surgery and are there either for the skin peel as an adjunct or for repair work.

The salon's beautician, Jacqueline Stallone, considers herself eminently qualified to comment on the subject and she does so quite joyously. Remember, she's partial to peeling.

"Plastic surgeons are frustrated butchers, crashing bores, and idiots," she says. "And please quote me accurately. They really belong in the undertaking business so they could not only bury their mistakes but bury the bodies as well. There really is a very fine line between undertakers and those doctors with sheepskins and scalpels.

"You should see some of the Ubangis that come in here. We get all the disasters of plastic surgery. The doctors tell them that having a facelift is no worse than going to a dentist. What they don't tell them is that their faces will fall down before their check clears.

"They have an uncanny knack of making one eye larger than the other, the better for peeking in keyholes. They always take too much out of the eyelids. One woman's bottom lid drooped down to her nose. . . . They're doing armpit lifts now, that's the latest. It's not a lift. It all falls down to the elbow. You get a tight armpit and a nice big plump elbow. . . .

"Some women are very stupid. They'll fall for anything if a doctor uses a little reverse psychology. He says, 'No, dear, you're not quite ready for a facelift. We'll just do a little nip-and-tuck, a mini-lift.' That sounds better, flatters them. And they wind up with the whole works, eyebrow lift, nose job, everything.

"The noses are the biggest disasters," she went on. "The doctor tells them they'll have a nice turned-up nose, then he smashes the bridge and they come out with a snoot. There's no way you can get any guarantees from plastic surgeons—except with busts. They'll line up the models for size and you pick out the ones you want. All the rest is potluck.

"Their hate and jealousy of each other is unbelievable. They're so money hungry some of them do three operations a day. That means they're on their feet twelve or fifteen hours. You can imagine what the last one they turn out looks like."

Jacqueline's unabashed disaffection for plastic surgeons is obviously colored by the fact that she's married to a face peeler. But even discounting her flair for the dramatic, and her woman's prerogative to exaggerate in making a point, it's a good point, one that should give people a lot of food for thought to chew on when they're thinking about a facelift and trying to decide—*Should I* or *Shouldn't I?*

Quite a few facelifted people out there will recognize themselves in this chapter, whether they've had their repair jobs done by Derma-Lift or the dozens or scores of plastic surgeons around the country who are also doing repair work on the botched-up jobs of other plastic surgeons.

Plastic surgeons, of course, are not the only kinds of surgeons who make mistakes. There was that terribly embarrassing mistake in a hospital in Philadelphia which made front-page headlines a while back and caused roars of chuckles in anti-medical circles, but it wasn't funny to the patients involved.

Two women were wheeled into surgery but, through a mixup, doctors got them confused and mistakenly started the operation that was intended for the other. Incisions had been made in the wrong places before the mistakes were discovered. One woman who had checked in with a ruptured disc had surgery for removal of a nodule from her parathyroid gland in the front of the neck, while the patient with the parathyroid problem underwent the initial stages of a cervical laminectomy at the back of her head.

If this can happen with specialists in ruptured discs and parathyroid glands, consider what your risks are with a facelift, which is much more common and more in demand.

The Nitty-gritty . . . This is the nitty-gritty of the risk problem in facelifts. There is a demand for plastic surgery. There are not enough qualified plastic surgeons to meet the demand. Plastic surgery lends itself to merchandising more than—well, how many demands are there for gall bladder operations? *The biggest risk for anyone seeking a facelift is landing in the hands of the wrong doctor.*

The Incompetents . . . With the boom in plastic surgery, there is also a boom in malpractice suits filed against the face-and-body lifters. Most of the doctors are not outright quacks or charlatans but bona fide licensed MDs who are merely incompetent at performing facelifts. The MD after their name makes it difficult for the unwary. Here's what can happen:

• Comedienne Totie Fields' physical troubles leading to a leg amputation and death began with a botched-up facelift. Her widower slammed a husband-wife doctor team with a $10,000 suit, charging they failed to warn Totie of the dangers of cosmetic surgery, and then failed to provide proper care after the operation, which he said contributed to her death. Totie was a diabetic, which undoubtedly had a great deal to do with her problems.

• In San Diego a "top flight" plastic surgeon, who had been frequently quoted as an "authority" in the press, was accused of "gross negligence and incompetence" in several civil actions filed against him by patients, through the state Board of Medical Quality Assurance.

According to the Board's accusation, the doctor performed breast surgery on one patient, removed an excess amount of nipple, placed the nipples too high, one higher than the other, and left her breasts with a "marked teardrop appearance." She won an $80,000 judgment against him. Another complaint involved a nose implant on a patient, which "came loose and moved to the right side of his nose." In still another, the complainant was a man who had undergone facelift surgery and was left with an unhealed wound across his forehead and a large abscess on the side of his neck. Also the doctor had removed so much skin from his lower eyelids that he would require "full-thickness skin grafts to correct the deformity," the complaint said.

Such gruesome examples are not chronicled here to alarm you, but to inform you that they do happen.

The Malcontents . . . At the other end of the pole are the patients who are simply malcontents, who are too picky for any plastic surgeon to please, and who switch doctors like musical chairs at the drop of a wrinkle. To be perfectly frank, I've seen a thousand per cent more lifted dimwits of this genre than the botched-up ones.

At a ladies luncheon in the Racquet Club one day I asked the ladies (for amusement and enlightenment) which of the plastic surgeons in Palm Springs they would choose if they wanted a facelift. All of them had already had at least two or three. The straw vote got sidetracked by an ex-liftee who leaned over the table, pulled back her hair, galvanized her index-finger tip upward behind her left earlobe, and said in a voice all choked up with fury, *"I* can tell you who *NOT* to go to. See this?"

Her finger was affixed on a small scar that couldn't have been seen by anyone without a magnifying glass until she pointed it out.

A friend of mine had her face done by one of the very high priests of the plastic surgeons' hierarchy (the ASPRS, American Society of Plastic and Reconstructive Surgeons), and was well satisfied for about six months. Then she noticed that a friend of hers who'd had a facelift from the same doctor was developing a pull at the corner of one eye and at one side of her mouth.

"I've decided that Dr. X operates on one side and a student on the other, because I'm seeing more and more of his work that is not quite symmetrical," she told me. She soon convinced herself that her own lift wasn't symmetrical and dashed off to Tahiti for a repair job.

I met a woman from Denver whose facelift was done by one of the leading plastic surgeons in that city. "Never again!"

she told me. "There were two of them working on me, one on one side of my face, another on the other side. I could hear them yakking through the anesthesia. They really botched me up. I'd never go through that again."

Within six months she'd had not only a new facelift but the complete bodyworks—breasts, thighs, tummy tucks, etcetera—by a Palm Springs Pygmalion she was ready to nominate for sainthood. Lord knows who's lifting her now.

As I said in the beginning, women are crazy. So we can't blame all the disasters on the doctors.

A New York plastic surgeon told me that he once had a patient on whom he did a rhinoplasty (nose job), and when she went home she was fine. Ten days later she came back; she had walked into a door and her nose was all pushed out of shape. The doctor redid it; she went home and ten days later she was back again. Same thing. She'd walked into a door. After two more instances of walking into a door and breaking her new nose, the doctor learned she was a drug addict.

Disaster Cases and Abuses . . . Though precise statistics are difficult to come by, it would appear to be a toss-up between Florida and California as to which is the largest—or most thriving—cosmetic surgery disaster center.

In Southern California especially, more reputable plastic surgeons have long been concerned about the situation. The Los Angeles *Times* and other newspapers have frequently carried long reports of medical surveys citing many cases of abuse in California. Typical are these summarized excerpts from a recent report:

• Spokesmen for the ASPRS of California say they are seeing increasing evidence that many doctors who are *unqualified* are busily at work in offices around the state.

• One Orange County plastic surgeon estimated that about 20 per cent of his practice is devoted to correcting the work of other doctors.

• One problem is *the same as in other states* (italics mine)—when a doctor receives a license to practice medicine, he is licensed as a "physician and surgeon," which means, according to a doctor on the ASPRS ethics committee, that *"you can do just about anything you want."*

• Medical experts say among the reasons cosmetic plastic surgery is attracting so many doctors is that it is fashionable and lucrative, and most of the procedures are elective and can be performed in the doctors' offices away from official observation.

• Board certified plastic surgeons say they are disturbed to find otolaryngologists (ENTs), dermatologists, and others performing breast surgeries, stomach tucks, and other procedures with little or no special training.

• The public (when seeking cosmetic surgery) should ascertain if the plastic surgeon is certified by the American Board of Plastic and Reconstructive Surgery.

• Certification by the Board means that a doctor, after completing his internship, has had a minimum of three years of general surgery training, a minimum of two additional years of training in plastic surgery, and has passed a written examination in the field. (The laws and regulations are rather uniform in most states; traditionally, doctors who practice specialties such as plastic surgery have devoted three to eight years of additional training *beyond* medical school.)

• One nurse was quoted in the report as saying that *very few doctors in Los Angeles are Board certified; they usually get their training from another doctor.*

• Dermatologists and otolaryngologists charged that, "The general plastic surgeon is only trying to protect his area because he feels someone will usurp him."

• Insurance companies with high malpractice insurance rates and high risk of lawsuits try to limit doctors to the things they do best. (But many plastic surgeons refuse to carry malpractice insurance, because it's too easy for facelift "malcontents" to sue them, merely on a whim, if they don't like their lift.)

• The survey found that the greatest abuses were going on in the offices of cosmetic surgery clinics and the private offices of doctors who work with cosmetic surgery referral services.

• Some plastic surgeons who have looked at problem cases say that "they are not exactly disasters but they are rather crudely done."

• One plastic surgeon told of a woman who had seven operations—five of them to correct errors.

• The greatest potential for unsatisfactory results is in cases handled by referral services.

• Typical mistakes (listed in the report) included such things as taking too much tissue from eyelids so that the patient's eyes remained open even when he or she went to sleep, and putting in breast implants that were too large, resulting in breasts with a poor appearance and eventually stretch marks.

• An officer of the Los Angeles Dermatological Society admitted that there are plastic surgery techniques in which dermatologists are not trained, but added, "A lot of dermatologists have gone back to school and brushed up on things."

• Organized plastic surgeons say that brush-up and other courses taken by doctors who are not certified plastic surgeons are inadequate preparation for a field like plastic surgery.

• Illustrations of "horror" stories in the report range from breasts ruined and noses botched to patients left with infections, pain, and aggravation.

These summarized excerpts, I repeat, are from a bona fide medical survey taken in Southern California. On the surface they would seem to confirm the observations made, but more colorfully expressed, by Jacqueline Stallone, the beautician in Miami.

Remove the label, and it's the same can of worms.

Now, if you're still interested in a facelift, read on.

13

The Big Hype

Why can't the laws and regulations prevent unqualified surgeons from operating?

First, as already mentioned and it should be emphasized, in the words of Dr. Peter Randall, a past president of the ASPRS:

"A physician licensed by state authority is legally entitled to practice in any field of medicine."

This in itself lets in many *licensed* but *unqualified* MDs to the lucrative practice of cosmetic surgery. It's the unqualified operators who are turning out most of the botched cases.

As one reputable plastic surgeon told me, "It's a sticky problem. In a free society, there is no way to control these people. The only solution is to inform the public."

The problem is compounded by what the more conservative doctors call, "The Big Hype."

In general, doctors have adhered to the rules of their national or state medical societies, which prevent members from advertising, whether or not they are prohibited by state law from soliciting patients.

However, many doctors who specialize in facelifts—whether plastic surgeons, dermatologists, or others—do not give two hoots about their national or state medical societies. Many of them are not even members of the AMA or their state medical society. They are not required to be.

If they're licensed, they can practice medicine.

Even many *Board certified* plastic surgeons are thumbing their bobbed noses at organized medicine, the AMA, their state medical society, and even the traditional academic hospital affiliation.

Many now have their own private clinics. The trend among facelifters is to flaunt all the rules of their peers in other branches of medicine. Dozens of licensed, Board certified doctors, mainly in California and Florida, proudly informed me that they didn't need affiliations with officially approved medical societies or hospitals. Some, in fact, have started their own non-officially approved "cosmetic surgery" societies of one kind or another.

As if this didn't cause enough problems already for the more legitimate and ethical physicians who are trying to maintain high medical standards within their own professional groups, now—enter Big Daddy, the government's Federal Trade Commission, which has opened the door to doctors' advertising.

In 1975, the FTC issued a complaint charging that medical societies were violating the law by preventing their members from advertising.

As this goes to press, the matter is under appeal and a final decision is still pending.

But a 1977 Supreme Court decision that sanctioned advertising by lawyers promptly set off a tornado of advertising by doctors—notably cosmetic surgeons.

And you simply wouldn't believe the way they're hawking their wares in California.

Full-page ads in the newspapers, hard-sell pitches on radio and TV, interviews on talk shows. . . . One Los Angeles plastic surgeon, a self-avowed egomaniac, has been on nearly every talk show in town, including a couple of sessions with Merv Griffin, talking about his wife's breasts and how he made them over—"So what. It's my wife and it's her breasts and if she wants to discuss them who am I to say no?"

He has been castigated by his fellow doctors, but he just shrugs and says, "They even say I have a PR firm. I don't but what's so terrible if I did? If I was a failure no one would care, but I think I have a certain amount of charm, I'm open, I speak in layman's terms, communicate, and have something called universal appeal. I happen to be one of the few bright spots as far as the public is concerned. They can identify with me. They need a folk hero among doctors. . . . I've been told privately that if I quieted down, in ten years I'd inherit the earth and be king of plastic surgery, but I am that already. Who's better known than I am? Nobody. I know I'm narcissistic, egomaniacal and neurotic, but I'm in control. You either like me or you don't."*

I wouldn't exactly put him on my A list but there are some who are gaga about him. I met a dazzling young girl at the last unveiling party I went to, who'd just had her nose done by him.

"How do you like it?" I asked.

"So-so," she said, with a little shrug. "It's dipped a little much." Pause. Faraway look in her eyes. Then, "But *HIM*. Wow! Those cowboy boots! He's *NEAT!*"

Since Him is so well known already, I do not feel obliged to use his name in this book.

If you want to identify with a folk hero, you're on your own.

His biggest competitor in the braggadocio end of facelifting is one who boldly and blatantly promotes his short-cut facelifts with beauty parlor techniques in his Sunset Boulevard pavilion.

"I do more surgery in a year then many do in a lifetime,"

* Ivor and Sally Davis, "New Faces For Everyone," *Los Angeles* magazine, April 1972.

he boasts. "I've taken facelifts from a four-hour procedure and two weeks in the hospital, down to twenty to thirty minutes—just like going to a dentist. With a breast enlargement, it's a five- to ten-minute thing and the woman can go out to the beach the same day and show off her new figure. I've fitted out the pavilion with a philosophy that surgery can be done with a beauty parlor technique, doing away with the hospital and having to put up with sick people groaning in the night."

Also, he points out, this does away with mammoth hospital bills.

"We feel people should visit their neighborhood plastic surgeon once every five years to keep in shape if they take pride in their appearance. After all, it takes less time to get rid of the wrinkles than to have their hair cut."

He has what he calls his forty-eight-hour beauty weekend. "Arrive Friday, have your nose bobbed, bags under eyes removed, wrinkles removed from face, size and firmness of breasts taken care of, and be home before the weekend is over."

This doctor is a licensed, Board certified plastic surgeon, not a member of any of the established professional medical societies. He has formed his own splinter group of "cosmetic plastic surgeons" and claims he has been trained under some of the best plastic surgeons in America. He has also written his own books as an "authority" on cosmetic surgery.

He isn't on my A list either, and if it's a forty-eight-hour beauty weekend you want with a beauty parlor technique for your facelift and bodyworks, this book isn't for you. You're still on your own.

Personally, I agree with the ASPRS position that the FTC Big-Daddy interference in a medical province already plagued with serious problems only adds to them further by encouraging advertising and opening the door wide to quickie merchants of cosmetic surgery.

The new breed of facelifters can now circumvent the accepted standards of quality and ethics by merely opening an office, running an ad campaign, and waiting for patients to come in for their cut-and-collect shenanigans.

And if they should happen to mutilate a few patients while learning their craft, they don't have to worry about the possibility of disciplinary action.

As one prominent plastic surgeon puts it, "The result of the government's sanction of advertising is that it only helps the unscrupulous."

Another explained, "The FTC maintains that we're restraining trade because we create only one product, one of excellence, and we limit our membership [ASPRS] based on stringent requirements for training. They're saying we've created artificially high standards. They're trying to tell us that *anybody who expresses an interest in plastic surgery must be admitted to our umbrella society* [ASPRS]. In other words, no longer are there qualifications of residency training and background, of standards, of examination—what they're saying is that anybody who walks up with a doctor's degree and says he's a plastic surgeon should be admitted—and should be permitted to advertise. And many now are doing it with the most flagrant forms of self-promotion."

To stem this tide the ASPRS of California itself launched an advertising campaign to warn the public of surgeons who advertise that they do plastic and reconstructive surgery but are not qualified to do so.

"The evidence we have thus far from California and several other states is that advertising is being used largely in a deceptive and misleading way by surgeons who are unqualified to do plastic and reconstructive procedures," the ASPRS stated.

The ASPRS's ad campaign to battle doctors' ads was confined to California because "that's where the problem is right now," said a spokesman who cited records of numerous cases where patients had responded with "disastrous" results to ads by unqualified surgeons.

"It is legal for any licensed physician to do plastic surgery —or any other kind of specialized surgery—even though he has not had specialty training," he said.

"Currently the AMA policy is that advertising for informational purposes is not unethical. The ASPRS believes that some California physicians go beyond the intent of the FTC or the AMA and mislead the patient and mis-state the physicians' qualifications . . .

"While the intent of the FTC opinion may have been to introduce competition and thus affect medical costs, we feel the welfare of the American patient is not well served by the way certain physicians have chosen to act under this new-found commercial freedom."

How does all of this affect *you?* It could affect you a great deal if you're seriously considering a facelift.

The Big Hype merchandising of cosmetic surgery is purely and simply a mirage.

And it is no longer confined only to California and Florida.

• In Chicago a lady lifter hawks her wares with "custom skin care and cosmetics" added to her plastic surgery armamentarium. She keeps lawyers busy with the suits filed against her and other doctors busy trying to undo what she's done.

• In Kansas City, a bastion of conservatism in cosmetic surgery, an enterprising young dude has come up with his own private-membership, country-club type Junior League for Liftees. For a $10,000 membership fee (family rate), you get all sorts of lifts plus consultations, a health-food smorgasbord, yoga lessons, and lots of other fringe benefits including a Gold Medallion with your name on one side and an engraved prayer on the other. The Jim Jones of the Lift Cult. He's a bona fide,

Board certified, licensed plastic surgeon, with the FTC's Gold Seal of approval for his Gold Medallion self-aggrandizing promotional brochures.

And if that's your bag, good luck.

14

The Big Con:
Before-and-After Photos

The Big Hype's stock-in-trade are the before-and-after photographs that bamboozle facelift candidates into thinking there's going to be a drastic difference in their faces.

Not true. If you have a homely face to begin with, no way will you come out looking like Elizabeth Taylor. The scalpel isn't a magic wand and doesn't perform miracles.

How much different you'll look with a new face depends on other things as well, mainly your hairdresser, your makeup, and the photographer or photographers who did your before-and-after pictures. Or, if you're a public figure, probably the photo editors who select them.

If you don't know how dreadful these people can make you look, just glance through almost any issue of the tabloid *National Enquirer*, whose photo editors seem to take special pleasure in using pictures that show entertainment celebrities and other well-known personalities at their worst.

Before-and-after facelift photos can and very often *do* lie. That old cliché that photographs don't lie, still accepted as gospel by those who want to believe it, simply is not true, as any professional photographer can tell you.

Betty Ford's facelift is a case in point. As I mentioned in an earlier chapter, the "before" photo of Mrs. Ford that was selected for syndication in newspapers and magazines must have been one of the most unflattering of her on file. Her "after" pictures did indeed show a dramatic change, due as much to her new hairstyle as the facelift. Millions of people were led to believe it was the lift alone that made the difference.

In fairness it should be pointed out that Mrs. Ford's plastic surgeon may have had nothing whatsoever to do with these before-and-after pictures. As a popular former First Lady, she is still very much in the public eye and constantly exposed to photographers' flashbulbs.

But the rip-off merchandisers of facelifting make flagrant use of before-and-after photos to lure the innocent into their lair.

In evaluating these photographs, it is important for you to know:

Photography can distort your face to look its best and worst with lights, shadows, and angles.

And many unethical facelifters hire photographers who specialize in this.

Technically it isn't at all difficult for a professional photographer who knows what he's doing. Before the operation he shoots you at an angle that gets the shadows in the right place until you look awful. After the operation, he drops the angle of the flash about 25 degrees, turns up the watts a few tenths, and your face turns out looking as though you're at a candlelight dinner.

At a medical meeting in Chicago, a photographer demonstrated with a patient how he could take before-and-after pictures to make her look as though she'd had a facelift even though she hadn't. He merely placed the patient on a tilt table, tilted her practically upside down, and photographed her from that angle. Then he turned her right-side up and shot another picture. When he developed the pictures he had a pair of perfect before-and-after shots for any facelifter's ads, brochures, or office come-on scrapbooks. The tilted patient looked as if she'd had a facelift, just because of the pull of gravity and the difference in the angles of the lights.

This is in no way meant to imply criticism of the legitimate use of medical photography by plastic surgeons. Quite the contrary. So far as I know, all plastic surgeons, even the most reputable and highly esteemed, do use photographs both as a record of their work (often for scientific papers and medical journals) and for discussions with their patients. In fact, most patients ask to see photographs, usually to help them understand what the doctor can do about their own special problems. And it is helpful to the doctors to have photographs so they can explain what can or cannot be done in certain areas —eyes, chin, nose, neck, and so on; and to answer patients' questions such as where the scars are going to be.

Most qualified doctors have at least two or three initial consultations with a patient. They have pictures made of the patient's face, then blown up on a viewer or projection screen so they can discuss certain details, and so both doctor and patient will have a better understanding of the problem.

But as one doctor explained, "Even under the best conditions, it's very difficult to get good medical photography. It should be done in a room set up for that purpose, with the light standardized in one location, with the same wattage each time, and the same angles. Only then can you make any approximate evaluation and comparison of the photographs."

Presumably, ethical doctors do not knowingly hire medical photographers who deliberately distort their pictures. But the very nature of photography itself, with its huge potential for accidentally or intentionally at least shading the truth, makes it an unpredictable tool in the medical kit and one of the greatest boons for the unscrupulous.

What it boils down to is that anyone, even without deliberate distortion, can pick the worst and the best of his before-and-after pictures to show to prospective facelift clients.

In the early days of plastic surgery, when it was still a new branch of medicine, many surgeons kept scrapbooks of photographs to show patients what could be accomplished. Over the years this custom fell into great disfavor for a very obvious reason. The scrapbooks showed only the good results, never the bad ones.

If a doctor does, say, one hundred facelifts and ninety-seven turn out to be flops and three turn out fine, which three do you think he's going to have in his scrapbook?

Ethical doctors do not use before-and-after photos as a sales pitch.

If a doctor hauls out a scrapbook to show you his good results, it's time to run.

Another trap in the facelift photo racket is the exploitation of celebrities. Their pictures are relatively easy to come by, especially those of movie stars and entertainment personalities. Some doctors' walls are plastered with pictures of famous people they have allegedly operated on.

At least three doctors in New York claim to have operated on the Duchess of Windsor.

Another New York plastic surgeon, who has performed many facelifts for celebrities in the social, theatrical, political, and diplomatic world, told me, "Most of these people do not want their pictures published or used in any way or under any circumstances whatever in connection with their operation. I happen to have an autographed picture of Mike Douglas, who is a friend of mine. I've never operated on Mike. I have another autographed picture of a famous movie star whom I have operated on. I could put both of them in my office but I don't. In the personal autographs, they're both glowing testimonials to me. They certainly would impress anyone who came in to my office—but one of them would be entirely fraudulent."

This doctor's advice on how to avoid being bamboozled by the Big Hype is:

• *Stay away from the doctor who prominently advertises his hospital connections (appointments are often political), his*

*membership in established medical societies (they don't guar-
antee a good operation), his roster of famous people he's
worked on; and avoid like poison the man who shows you a
scrapbook of good results.*

15

The Big Controversy:
Hospital or Office Surgery

The newest trend and most heated topic of controversy in cosmetic surgery does not involve medical techniques but rather the whereabouts of the operation.

There's a big boom in doctors' office surgery. As usual, it started in California but is rapidly expanding to other states. And as usual in this branch of medicine, it has its fiercely virulent and vocal boosters and detractors.

The boosters say they're saving patients thousands of dollars, avoiding hospital red tape and bureaucracy, and providing high quality medical service at a comparatively low cost.

The detractors say that too many office surgeons are unqualified or incompetent; that deaths, injuries, and other complications are occurring in increasing numbers; that a doctor's private office should not be used as an operating room because it isn't subject to inspection or licensing by a public health agency.

The situation is confused and chaotic for anyone contemplating a facelift.

I suggest that you digest these chapters carefully before making your decision.

Surveys indicate that between 50 and 85 per cent of all doctors performing plastic surgery in California do it in their offices; some experts contend that about the same percentage applies nationwide, and this doesn't include doctors doing plastic surgery who are not plastic surgeons.

Dr. John Williams of Beverly Hills, one of the pioneers of the office-surgery movement, says the boom started because of new office-surgery techniques widely reported in medical journals and a concerted effort to control costs.

"Unfortunately," he adds, "it's the perfect setup for someone who's unqualified. They are totally freewheeling, unsupervised, unrestrained in what they do."

Office surgery is more convenient for both doctor and patient; it eliminates a lot of paperwork that hospitals require; and in Dr. Williams's opinion, "This is all right, largely, because we're operating basically on well people."

Doctors say the average cost of cosmetic surgery done in the office is about one third of the same thing done in a hospital.

"The people who abuse something will do so regardless of the license requirements. California is a prime example. You've got people doing plastic surgery in California who don't even know what it is," said an ASPRS spokesman in Miami.

A Los Angeles *Times* inquiry into the office-surgery situation in November 1979 found that:

• Though hundreds of California surgeons operate in their offices, there is no mandatory system to make certain they are competent to perform the operations they offer. Even if they have been stripped of hospital surgical privileges for incompetency, or denied them in the first place for lack of training, their office operating practices are completely unrestricted.

• Deaths from in-office operations occur frequently, though most experts agree office surgery should be performed only on the healthiest of patients. Death reports reach the Los Angeles County Medical Examiner's office at the rate of one every six to eight weeks. "That's a helluva lot," said one deputy medical examiner.

Because many office-surgery deaths involve patients never sent to the hospital, investigators believe that a "substantial" number escape detection entirely because the doctors involved issue the death certificates themselves.

• Ear, nose, and throat specialists, urologists, and even dermatologists have started to cash in on the office-surgery boom, attempting operations like repositioning belly buttons and increasing or reducing the size of women's breasts. (At the time of this report, a Sacramento urologist was facing criminal charges in such a case.)

• Though there have been deaths, blindings, cripplings, and other doctors' office catastrophes in recent years, no city, county, state, or federal agency is seeking power to regulate office surgery. Doctors' associations believe such mandatory enforcement will inevitably be inaugurated unless office surgeons do a better job of policing themselves.

"This isn't the kind of thing surgeons have always done in their offices," said one top surgeon. "Surgeons have always routinely done mole removals, cysts, and things like that in the back room using Novocain, but this is different. A lot of this is major surgery."

And it can sometimes amount to an invitation to tragedy.

• One such tragedy occurred in the office of Dr. G., a *Board certified* plastic surgeon, meaning he had passed a test on his skills given by other plastic surgeons. He did a rhinoplasty (nose surgery) on Jeff S., seventeen, a high school graduation gift from his parents. Nine days later he was dead. The catastrophic complications that led to the youth's death do not need to be chronicled here. Whether his death was due to a "freak drug reaction" or blood running down his windpipe and into his lungs, as various medical reports stated, probably no one really knows. The death certificate called the case a "therapeutic accident."

It may be years before a court rules who—if anyone—was at fault in Jeff's death. But the case was far from the first incident of serious complications during office surgery. Some past cases have resulted in criminal and civil court action. Others are in litigation as this is being written. Still more are under investigation by the California State Board of Medical Quality Assurance—and investigative Board counterparts in other states.

• Office surgery involving general anesthesia is being widely done in Miami, Houston, Chicago, New York, and other major population areas.

Lawyers and doctors familiar with office surgery say unqualified *physicians who advertise their services experience the highest rates of complications* (italics mine).

One case that received wide public attention involved an Orange County *Board certified* plastic surgeon charged with the death of a woman in his Santa Ana office during a breast implant operation. He was one of Southern California's most heavily advertised plastic surgeons. Originally, a death certificate branded the fatality as only an "accident." The surgeon was charged with murder in a multicount indictment. (For details, see next chapter.)

Jean S., fifty-nine, went to the office of Palm Springs plastic surgeon Dr. T. for a facelift. She made reservations to stay at a hotel near the doctor's office. Before the surgery, she gave him $4,000 in full payment for his fee. According to depositions in a malpractice suit filed against the doctor, the operation progressed without incident in the office.

But when the sedated Mrs. S. returned to her hotel room, she complained of intense pain in her left eye. Her son called the doctor's office but did not reach him. Instead, his nurse was dispatched to the hotel to examine the bandages and patches over both eyes. (Author's note: I personally know of *too many* cases where the doctor could not be reached and some sort of "nurse" or flunky was sent for the follow-up.)

The nurse allegedly concluded the dressings looked normal, but that evening Mrs. S. complained of sudden bleeding from the left eye. The doctor did not have office hours the following day, and Mrs. S. was again seen by the nurse who said everything was still "normal."

Twenty-four hours later, when the doctor removed the patches, he discovered that Mrs. S. was blind in her left eye.

The doctor contended (through his attorney) that the blinding was an "unavoidable complication," and that the loss of vision could not have been prevented if Mrs. S. was in a hospital room instead of the hotel. The case has not yet been resolved.

The Los Angeles *Times* inquiry also found that:

• An increasing number of ENT specialists are branching out into breast reconstruction plastic surgery, frequently with disastrous results. In almost every case, the physicians are doing breast reductions or enlargements in their offices even though few reputable hospitals would permit them to do such operations because they are not trained to perform them.

• One malpractice suit involved a San Fernando Valley physician who allegedly botched a facelift operation he was performing in a hospital, and then tried to repair the damage in a procedure in his office. During the second operation, the woman, who had a history of heart trouble, suffered a near-fatal heart attack. A third surgery was required to enable her to close her eyes again normally.

Some medical organizations are working toward state laws and regulations to bring the doctors' office operating rooms within somewhat the same requirements and standards as a hospital. But again, as usual, this move is met with heavy resistance by most of organized medicine, including the AMA (as well as the California Medical Association, the Los Angeles County Medical Association, etcetera, etcetera, etcetera), whose lobbyists contend that licensing or inspecting a doctor's office would interfere with the doctor's right to practice his profession, and thus would strike at the heart of his right to run his own business under the free enterprise system.

So they are outside the authority of any health agency. When health inspectors come, it's only to check on the restaurant in the building's lobby level.

• Though accidents and cover-ups by doctors occur in hospitals, too, most health centers have internal regulatory committees that constantly review the surgeons' operating rooms. While such actions are almost never publicly acknowledged, hospital surgical committees frequently vote to strip individual surgeons of the right to perform certain operations.

• Some physician groups have opened so-called "surgicenters," large independent clinics that perform outpatient surgery but which are not part of a hospital. The surgical centers, however, must meet state licensing standards that apply to clinics and gain accreditation from one of two national health-facility certification groups. (There are ten accredited surgical centers in California.)

• The American Society of Plastic and Reconstructive Surgeons, with headquarters in Chicago, has formed a committee to push for "suggested standards" for doctors' operating rooms. Chairman of the committee is Dr. Paul Pickering, a prominent plastic surgeon in San Diego. But his set of "suggested standards" has drawn criticism from California plastic surgeons who complain that the rules are too restrictive and costly to implement. Experts have agreed that few office operating rooms could pass muster. Among the standards:

• Operating rooms must be at least nine by twelve feet, with a well-designed operating table, good lighting, and a backup electrical system in case power in the building goes out. (Hospital surgical suites commonly have emergency generators.)

• A full range of emergency medical equipment must be on hand with backup systems for each piece of equipment in case of failure. There must be a "crash cart" as well equipped as that found in any major hospital emergency room.

• There must be two oxygen-supply systems and each operating room must be staffed by a qualified anesthesiologist any time a general anesthetic is to be used.

• Every employee of the office practice must be qualified to administer cardiopulmonary resuscitation—including secretaries, file clerks, and receptionists.

• A full-time registered nurse must be employed to run the surgical facility. All equipment must be inspected daily.

"The way it is now," Dr. Pickering said, "if the guy's got an MD he can hang you in his office."

His suggested standard program could become part of a formal accrediting process nationwide, administered by members of the ASPRS; and each office operating suite would be inspected by a committee of surgeons.

In the over-all picture of cosmetic surgery in this country, and at the rate plastic surgeons and everyone else doing plastic surgery are arguing among themselves, my personal guess is that it may be quite a while before anyone gets around to drawing up a code of standards and ethics that can be enforced on doctors doing cosmetic operations in their offices.

In the majority of cases, as most doctors agree, the operations turn out just as well (or as badly) as they would have if performed in a hospital.

The main problem is *IF* something goes wrong, *IF* you have a stroke, or a heart attack, or any other serious complications during your facelift in a doctor's office, is the doctor equipped to handle such emergencies or can he get you to the hospital in time?

It's a big IF.

In the case of Kim Plock, thirty-three, something did go wrong in the doctor's office, and the doctor was charged with murder. . . . Don't let it happen to you. . . . Read on.

16

The Big Question . . .

Who Is Qualified to Perform Plastic Surgery— and Who Decides?

One of the most notorious malpractice cases in Southern California has achieved widespread nationwide publicity because of its far-reaching implications in the significant and growing problems of plastic surgery.

It underscores the fundamental issue of *who is a plastic surgeon?* It encapsulates the conflict between the plastic surgery profession and the Federal Trade Commission. It epitomizes with well-documented gory details what *can* happen to *you* if you land in the hands of the wrong doctor.

The central character in this scenario is a young licensed MD who enjoyed a short but checkered foray in private practice as a self-styled plastic surgeon. He had the distinction of being one of Southern California's most heavily advertised surgeons. He operated in his office. He called his office the "Doctor's Plastic Surgery Medical Group."

He was only in business a little more than a year but in that short time he became embroiled in far more trouble than most doctors face in a lifetime—with seventeen malpractice suits and a long list of criminal charges filed against him, including murder.

Dr. Ralph J. W. Small is out of jail now, after serving only ninety days, and by the time this is in print he may have hung up his shingle again. He is still licensed to practice—as an ENT doctor.

The criminal charges alleged that in addition to the death of one patient, others were maimed.

The most publicized case involved the death of thirty-three-year-old Kim Plock, a woman on whom Small was performing a breast-reduction operation in November 1978. Investigators (for the Board of Medical Quality Assurance) later found that an *unlicensed* medical technician employed by Dr. Small had administered a dangerously large dose of an anesthetic called Innovar to Mrs. Plock. She lapsed into a coma, Small tried to revive her, then sent an employee to another doctor's office in the same building to ask if he could borrow a tank of oxygen. Eventually, after *nine hours* of working on her, he called an ambulance to hospitalize her. But since he was not a member of the hospital staff, he was barred from looking at her medical chart during the five days before she died.

The unlicensed technician who administered the anesthesia later pleaded guilty to practicing medicine without a license. The charges against Small were more numerous—a forty-one-count complaint in an eleven-page allegation, which also included charges of grand theft for taking patients' money under false pretenses—i.e., telling them he was a Board certified plastic surgeon when he had completed less than six months of training in the field.

The original multicount murder indictment was changed to manslaughter after some legal plea-bargaining negotiations; Small would plead guilty to the manslaughter charge in exchange for the state's dropping all the other counts.

Actually, the criminal trial was never held. Small was sent off for a ninety-day "pre-sentence evaluation" in the state prison at Chino, then released on probation.

Small practiced in Santa Ana, California. Dr. Robert

Miner, president of the Orange County (in which Santa Ana is located) Society of Plastic Surgeons, and other Orange County physicians who were prepared to testify against Small at the criminal trial that was never held were flabbergasted.

Said Dr. Miner, "As far as the Orange County plastic surgeons are concerned, they are upset because they feel that in all the time they've been in practice, they've never come across something that was so blatantly wrong.

"We felt that here's a guy who has done the worst . . . and the legal system is saying, 'Doctors, heal yourself. Clean your own house.'

"We go to bat and say this guy should never be allowed to practice that kind of medicine again and the court turns around and sends him right back to us."

According to court records and affidavits, Dr. Small's key contention was that he was singled out for persecution by his colleagues because he believes in physician advertising.

He also contended that the appellation "Board certified," meaning a doctor had passed a minimum competency test in his specialty, was "meaningless" and that the American Board of Plastic Surgery was nothing more than a "social club."

Dr. Miner's response to this was, "We're not mad at him because he advertised or because he did things in his office that he didn't know anything about. We're mad because of the way he behaved in treating the welfare of his patients. I've got a dozen patients of his who have to go back into surgery, and in the newspapers and on TV he's saying, 'I'll be back doing plastic surgery.'

"We're upset at the ease with which someone can call himself a plastic surgeon, regardless of his background. You have to have some sort of minimum standards. But I don't know how you're going to stop it [increasing malpractice] now. We have so many laws to protect people that it's almost impossible to get someone who's flagrantly guilty out of practice."

Among the most flagrant of the malpractice cases among Dr. Small's patients who landed in Dr. Miner's hands was one that in his opinion is more medically significant than the Plock death, which got most of the headlines.

It involved an attempted thigh-lift operation, a procedure to smooth skin wrinkles on the thighs and buttocks. Dr. Small had never attempted the operation before. In fact, he had only read a single medical journal article about it before he tried the operation on Marcia Weed.

It is an operation which even few practitioners experienced in doing it would attempt in their offices.

But Dr. Small did.

When Ms. Weed came out of the anesthetic, she complained of pain in her legs. Small told her there was no serious problem, but he kept her in the office overnight; then he led her to his van the next day, had her lie down on the floor of the vehicle because she could not stand, and drove her home.

The complications worsened. The tissue around the incisions turned a dark color. The doctor decided on further surgery. Ms. Weed returned to Small's office.

This time, she stayed in the suite for five days. Small said it was her choice. He said he told her he could hospitalize her —though he did not have admitting privileges at any hospital —or keep her in the office. He said he advised her that staying in his office would be cheaper since he had already collected an all-inclusive fee for surgery—$3,025.

During the stay, office employees brought take-out fast food to Ms. Weed.

Finally, the doctor took her home again, leaving her with instructions to wash off the affected areas of her legs.

Eventually, Ms. Weed sought other medical assistance. Her case was *diagnosed as gangrene* and she suffered deep erosion of the tissue in her thighs. As this is written, she is still undergoing treatment to try to reconstruct her legs, more than a year after her botched-up thigh-lift.

At least she survived.

She has had two operations to correct the damage, which could have been fatal.

"She is coming along well," Dr. Miner told me.

But he wasn't hesitant about expressing the bitterness that many doctors feel, not necessarily toward Dr. Small himself but toward the system that let him and his patients end up where they did.

A capsule look at Dr. Small's medical background and practices provides, in my opinion, an excellent insight into why many people are bamboozled into cosmetic surgery con-traps.

It isn't all your fault. You're dealing with some of the world's neediest-greediest medical swindlers with sometimes the most impeccable credentials.

A prime example is Dr. Ralph J. W. Small, whose career was temporarily interrupted by the foregoing, highly publicized "irregularities" before the age of thirty-two. Yet, when he was a student at the famed Bronx High School of Science in New York City, he was considered a boy genius. The trouble was he didn't use his genius in the right direction, though his early academic indoctrination was most impressive. He was admitted to the prestigious Massachusetts Institute of Technology, then to the medical school at Johns Hopkins University, and did his internship at the University of Michigan Hospital in Ann Arbor.

You can't get more impressive than all of that.

Then, in July of 1971, Ralph Small arrived at the University of California Medical Center in San Francisco for the first year of a residency in *brain surgery*. And the first of the lingering questions emerged.

He resigned abruptly from the brain surgery program in 1972, a year after he entered it. Court documents indicate he was advised to resign or face firing. Somehow he gained a position as a resident in ear, nose, and throat medicine at the University of California Irvine Medical Center. He completed the program, eventually gaining Board certification in that narrow specialty. Then it was discovered that his letters of recommendation from San Francisco had been "forged with intent to defraud."

There was a small flurry of academic-legal-medical hassling which no one outside that sphere can presume to comprehend; but the upshot was that Small set up shop in Santa Ana and heavily advertised himself as a plastic surgeon, though he had completed less than six months of the two years' training required for the specialty. Strangely, the UC Irvine faculty had made no public complaint, and prosecutors reportedly did not know of either the San Francisco or Irvine situations when the plea bargaining was going on.

The Small case has opened up—again—the continuing, deep-seated controversy over just how far ear, nose, and throat doctors can legitimately go into plastic surgery. And that bone of contention, experts agree, may eventually turn out to be more important than Small as an individual.

Ear, nose, and throat specialists—or otolaryngologists—observe a de facto border on the body. *They do not perform surgery on organs below the shoulders.*

Few reputable hospitals will allow an ENT to perform such surgery—unless, like only about thirty-five physicians nationwide—he has earned specialty Board certification in plastic surgery too.

Dr. Mark Krugman of Tustin, California, is one of the few Board certified ENT-plastic surgeons in practice anywhere in the country. Because he has background in both fields of medicine, Krugman said he was especially incensed at what happened in the Small case. He, too, was one of the Orange County doctors who went to court to testify in a preliminary hearing in the Small criminal case.

"This situation represents a larger thing than Small," he said. "It is the futility of our fight with the Federal Trade Commission."

He was referring to the FTC's stand that the plastic surgery board's membership standards are too strict and that by preventing doctors who want to perform plastic surgery from doing so, the Board is engaged in restraint of trade.

Plastic surgeons mobilized, spending nearly $1 million in legal fees to force the FTC to listen to their case: That Board certification is a necessary guarantee for consumers that doctors are minimally competent.

As this is written, the FTC's investigation of the plastic surgery board is still going on.

And Ralph Small is still at liberty.

Author's Note: Large portions of the last two chapters were condensed and reprinted by special permission of the Los Angeles *Times* from two feature articles by *Times* staff writer Allan Parachini:

"THE BOOM IN DOCTORS' OFFICE
   SURGERY," November 11, 1979
"JAILED SURGEON: NEW QUESTIONS
   RAISED," November 28, 1979

17

The Doctors:

Telling It Like It Is

I have purposely focused in previous chapters on a situation in Southern California because:

1. It involves flagrant abuses that have been thoroughly investigated and documented by many independent investigators other than myself.

2. It reflects and reinforces certain findings and conclusions from my own research and interviews.

3. It has been brought to the public's attention in California but I feel it should be brought to public attention on a nationwide scale.

4. It includes practices, procedures, and questions that should be of vital concern and could have grave implications not only for the entire medical profession but for the public as well.

Readers of this book especially should give thoughtful consideration to such questions as whether a doctor is qualified to perform plastic surgery, whether he is equipped to operate in his office—and why it is necessary for him to advertise.

Dr. Robert Miner, president of the Orange County Society of Plastic Surgeons, and the surgeon who inherited most of Dr. Small's botched cases, summed it up for me in an interview, and his remarks may come as a surprise to many.

"The trouble is, we have more doctors than we need and they're hungry. They're looking for business," he said. "So they are widening the scope of the things they do, and they're widening the scope beyond their training. This is going to become more and more apparent in the future.

"The basic problem is that any licensed MD can practice plastic surgery if he wants to. This is true in all states. It's difficult to get any legislation passed to restrain them because this would be for the benefit of specialists and the majority of doctors are general practitioners who don't want legislation to benefit specialists.

"Also, for years the public has been led to believe that we don't have enough doctors to take care of sick people. This simply isn't true. Instead of too few, we have too many. They need patients, they need money, so they're doing facelifts. All residency programs are turning out more and more plastic surgeons. More than 50 per cent of the plastic surgeons now practicing have only started in the past five years because of the boom in facelifts. The schools keep turning out more and more, and everybody's getting hungry.

"There is an overabundance of specialists of all kinds without any great abundance of patients for their specialties. Plastic surgeons, for instance, are trained in reconstructive surgery—for things like burns, injuries, birth defects, cleft palates. There's no overabundance of cleft palates, but there's a great abundance of people wanting cosmetic surgery and it's very lucrative. That's why so many people are getting into the act. This is money up front. It doesn't have to pass through the books. A lot of doctors take it under the table."

Dr. Miner said there is a special problem with the ENT doctors that has caused their intrusion into plastic surgery.

"The ENT specialty is going through a great transition period," he explained, "because many of the things the otolaryngologists specialized in have simply disappeared with new medical techniques and antibiotics. The ENT men used to do a lot of tonsil surgery, sinus surgery, inner ear surgery. Antibiotics now take care of some of these problems. There's not so much demand today for an ENT specialist. Antibiotics have almost wiped out that specialty; the ENT men have to look for new horizons so they start doing facelifts. One does it and the next one says, 'If he can do it, I can too.' But they don't even stop at faces, they do operations on breasts and abdomens.

"And there's no law that stops them. As long as they have a license to practice medicine, they can do anything, according to the FTC. What it boils down to is that most of the abuses in cosmetic surgery are really supported by our government."

Advertising: The Big Sham . . .

Dr. Miner's views on doctor advertising are harsh, outspoken, logical, and enlightening to anyone considering a facelift. Read them carefully. He says:

"Ask yourself these questions: Why does a doctor advertise? A doctor advertises to get patients. Why can't he get patients in the regular fashion? If he is not getting patients, why not?

"There must be a reason why he is not getting patients and the reason is either that he does poor work or he is not what he claims to be. In most cases he's a schlock with a sham operation. From the ads you think you're getting a bargain; the fees for his facelifts are cheaper. But have you ever stopped to think about what the ads cost him? He has to boost his practice up enough to pay for his advertising so he promises you the moon and cuts costs by cutting down on quality. He hauls in patients with his ad baits, runs them through like a Sears and Roebuck operation, and they don't get it done the way it should be done, so they go back and have it done every year because all they got was a little tuck, not a facelift. *It's a sham operation*. They've never really had a facelift. That little tuck costs a lot of money and he makes a lot of money because when the swelling goes down and the wrinkles come back, the patients come back, and he tells them, 'You're one of those poor people with the type of skin where the wrinkles come back fast.' The people don't know the difference, they take his word for it. When their faces flop they just assume they're one of those poor unfortunates that can't get it tight.

"It wasn't done right in the first place."

The only reason there aren't more serious injuries in such sham operations, Dr. Miner explained, is that, "There is very little done and therefore very little risk. A little tuck here and there isn't difficult to do. When you stop to think about it, probably 50 per cent of all babies born could be delivered by cab drivers.

"But if you're going to have a baby, you don't stop at a cab stand. If the public would bother to check out the credentials and qualifications of the doctors who advertise facelifts, a lot of these hungry schlocks would die of malnutrition. We're doing all we can to get these people off the streets. It's up to the public to help us by being informed and not patronizing them.

"There are plenty of legitimate, highly qualified plastic surgeons. I'm amazed at the casual way some people decide on a doctor to do their facelifts. They don't spend as much time and thought on picking a surgeon as they do on picking a new automobile. It's absurd."

As for performing surgery in the office or hospital, Dr. Miner does both. "It depends on the operation," he said. "If a doctor is qualified and his office is well staffed and equipped, there is no reason not to perform facelifts in the office. More and more legitimate plastic surgeons are doing it. The risks and complications are very rare when they are performed by qualified surgeons."

But, he warned, if you choose to have your facelift done in an office, be sure to go to a doctor affiliated with a hospital.

"The big difference between a legitimate plastic surgeon

and a schlock," he said, "is that one is qualified to do the operation in the hospital as well as the office, and the other is not."

Following are summaries of interviews on this subject with two of the nation's most prominent plastic surgeons, one in Chicago and the other in New York.

Dr. Peter McKinney, Associate Professor of Plastic Surgery at Northwestern University Medical School, former president of the Chicago Society of Plastic Surgery.

• "There is still a great deal of guilt and secrecy surrounding cosmetic surgery and that's why it started in offices, really, before it moved into medical centers. Plastic surgery was always respected when we talked about burns, cleft palates, congenital anomalies—but when we talked about facelifts or things of this nature, we were sometimes isolated and ridiculed by our peers as catering to vanity. Many patients also were subjected to the same prejudice. They felt guilty for taking up a doctor's time and a hospital bed when there were really sick people all around them. I think the role of cosmetic surgery is changing. We have a very healthy relationship here, with the university. I feel less of the prejudice here than in the East, but I think it still exists to some extent. I'm sure some of us still sense a certain attitude in certain people—as though they're thinking, 'Hmmmmm, doing another facelift . . . dealing in that frivolous matter.'

"I do no surgery in the office; it's all in the hospital. But I think it makes absolutely no difference if you have optimum conditions, adequate backup in case of a problem.

"Remember, THIS IS MAJOR SURGERY; IT'S NOT GETTING A JACKET TAILORED. If you have proper support and sterility and so forth, the location doesn't make any difference. You could set up an office to do it just as well as in a hospital.

"There are doctors in Chicago who perform surgeries in their offices. Not all of them have optimum conditions, but some do."

Many who, like Dr. McKinney, are affiliated with prestigious medical centers and have close relationships with university hospitals, simply prefer to perform their surgery in the hospital rather than incur the expense of installing operating facilities in their offices.

Dr. McKinney also is very much opposed to the government's ruling that permits physicians to advertise. "It only helps the unscrupulous," he said. As for the FTC's "restraint of trade" stance on the ASPRS, he feels that it is an attempt to open up the membership so that anyone who holds an MD diploma could become a member of the ASPRS.

He has very strong feelings on the big hype and merchandising of cosmetic surgery by unqualified practitioners, which, like Dr. Miner and others, he believes is being supported and encouraged by the government.

And like Dr. Miner, he feels it's up to the public to be informed and wary. "Let the public be the judge," he says. "It's really *caveat emptor*. Let the buyer [the patient] beware. Some people *want* snake oil. But maybe only about 10 per cent of the population. The crux of this kind of merchandising is very much related to the whole idea of giving people false hopes, as well as abbreviated information. If you buy a toaster and decide you don't want it, you can return it. If you get a bad result with a face, it can't always be fixed—and you can't return it."

Dr. Thomas D. Rees, MD, FACS, Associate Professor of Clinical (Plastic) Surgery, New York University; Attending Surgeon, Plastic Surgery, Manhattan Eye, Ear and Throat Hospital, New York, New York.

• "The choice of whether to operate in a hospital, in a clinic, or in the office is very much an individual question. Of course, the main prerequisite is that the operating room conditions are adequate to handle any and all emergency exigencies which may occur, so that the patient is afforded maximum safety. Many surgeons in the U.S. have excellent outpatient ambulatory surgical clinics in association with their office or a related facility. I personally prefer to do major operations in the hospital. I insist on hospital surgery for those patients which have any medical condition indicating that the risk assumed in elective surgery is slightly or significantly more than that in a so-called 'normal patient.'

"We have an excellent outpatient surgical ambulatory facility in our office, complete with operating rooms and recovery room. I prefer to operate on the patient who is in good medical condition, and where the patient feels most comfortable. Many patients feel threatened by a hospital atmosphere and do much better in an outpatient clinic, where they are allowed to go home. The patient has a choice under these conditions.

"Also, in some instances and in many states, third party insurance coverers do not cover the hospital costs for elective plastic surgery and these patients can save a good deal of money by being operated upon in an outpatient facility where the costs to the patient are much less.

"Once again, it is the safety of the patient that is our primary concern and those patients which have any questionable medical conditions should be operated upon in the hospital.

"I do give my patients the option of being operated upon in my outpatient surgical clinic or in the hospital, provided there are no medical surgical conditions contraindicating outpatient clinic surgery.

"I do maintain a very well equipped outpatient facility, along with an excellently trained staff.

"I use either a local or general anesthetic, again according to the patient's desire. However, I do insist on a general anesthetic with a highly trained expert anesthetist for any patient with a coexisting medical condition such as a history of heart disease, diabetes, allergies to local anesthetic, and so forth."

18

Straight from the Mouth of the Top Banana

In the preparation of this book, I have been warned repeatedly by the most eminently qualified plastic surgeons that I should use the utmost caution in my choice of doctors to interview and quote.

Among the golden nuggets of advice given to me by each eminently qualified plastic surgeon is to steer clear of that other eminently qualified Dr. So-and-so because he's either too old-fashioned, far-out, or doesn't know from borscht.

My golden-nugget collectibles of scalpel swipes among the eminently qualified So-and-sos would fill another whole book. But once around is enough.

Personally, my biggest disillusionment in this project has been the discovery of a morass of brotherly knife-stabs at each other; and frankly, my biggest reason for balking at a facelift is not for fear they'll cut up my face but for a strong allergy to anyone in any profession whose members are so bent on cutting up one another.

It is not, in my opinion, a very pretty commentary on a

profession that has so much to do with making our faces prettier.

I have chosen to include in this book the fact sheet of an eminently qualified plastic surgeon in New York, Dr. Thomas D. Rees, because I happen to think it is the best of all roundup advice I've seen printed for facelift candidates.

Dr. Rees gives the printed fact sheets to all his facelift patients. (He gives a different set to those wanting nose jobs.)

He has been known for years as one of the world's leading plastic surgeons; and if all of you other eminently qualified plastic surgeons want to argue about it, that's your problem.

Once again, this is not a personal recommendation. (He probably couldn't book you for years anyway.) However, his concise summary of facts is one which everyone should read and think about before deciding on whether to have a facelift.

SOME FACTS FOR PATIENTS ABOUT COSMETIC FACIAL AND EYELID SURGERY

You will do yourself a service if you read what follows carefully, for here you will find answers to many of the questions that are most often asked about plastic surgery of the face, neck and eyelids. Most of these questions are universally asked by patients interested in this type of surgical correction.

The purpose of cosmetic surgery is to make you look as good as it is possible for you to look. It cannot do more than that. If you are expecting a transforming miracle from surgery, you will unquestionably be disappointed. Plastic surgery is a combination of art and science. Surgery is altogether not an exact science, and because some of the factors involved in producing the final result (such as the healing process) are not entirely within the control of either the surgeon or patient, it is impossible to warranty or guarantee results. Surgical results from facial and eyelid plastic surgery, however, are more predictable in some patients than others. This is determined by a number of factors such as the physical condition of the face, the thickness and condition of the skin, the presence or absence of facial fat, the relative "age" of the skin, the numbers and types of wrinkles present, the underlying bone structure, heredity and hormonal influences, and others.

It is not possible, by surgical operation, to make someone who is over forty years old look as if he or she is twenty years old or younger! While this may seem obvious, I mention it because some patients through misconceptions or misinformation believe the clock can be turned back in this miraculous fashion. It cannot.

Surgery intended to improve sagging skin or wrinkles necessarily leaves scars. Despite what you may have heard, all surgical scars are permanent and cannot be erased. The job of the plastic surgeon is to place scars in natural lines of the face and eyelids, where they are least noticeable and are more easily camouflaged by make-up or hair styles. While such scars are permanent, they are rarely noticeable or cause any trouble.

(1) How long will the surgical results last?

Plastic surgery of the face, neck and eyelids retards the aging process and actually slows it up. It "slows down the clock, but does not stop it." It is not a question of a sudden "falling down." How soon you will want, or require another operation is highly individualized. I can only speak in averages. In general, the operation of facial and neck lift, which is for the improvement of the jowls along the jaw line and the loose skin of the neck, may need to be redone in about five to eight years. Some very few patients are encountered who, for one reason or another, age more rapidly so that another operation may be desired in a shorter period of time than five years. Of course there are some who never require it again. The operation to improve or correct "bags" of the eyelids usually lasts longer. In most instances the pouches beneath the lower lids do not recur. As one grows older the skin becomes looser and redundant and a trim of loose skin may be necessary at a later time. In those patients where there is exceedingly marked aging and excessive skin of the neck, face and jaw, sometimes (but extremely rarely), it is necessary to perform a second operation within a year to achieve the maximum improvement possible. If this seems to be the situation in your case, I will so inform you in advance.

(2) Can complications occur from cosmetic facial surgery?

Complications can occur from any type of surgery. They cannot be anticipated in cosmetic facial surgery, but are most often minor in nature. The most common complication after a face lift or eyelid surgery is hematoma. A hematoma is a collection of blood under the skin. In about 2% of all face lift operations this collection of blood must be removed in the immediate postoperative period. Small hematomas are simply removed and treated several days after surgery as an outpatient procedure. Such complications as nerve paralysis, infection, eye irritation, skin ulceration, scar over-growth (a keloid) and so forth also can occur—but rarely. These and other obscure complications will be discussed with you in detail if you so desire. It is my duty to inform you of the possibility of these complications not to alarm or frighten you, but as a point of information.

(3) Why are preoperative photographs important?

Just as the chest surgeon cannot operate in an intelligent way without x-rays of the chest, the plastic surgeon cannot operate on the face or eyelids without medical photographs. These photographs are not meant to flatter you. You probably will find it a harsh photograph unsuitable for framing. The photographs show your face in every detail. This aids greatly in the surgical performance of technical variations in the surgery.

(4) What type of anesthesia is used during the operation?

Either local or general anesthesia can be used, according to preference. I prefer to use a combination of light general anesthesia and local anesthesia, which I find is more comfortable for the patient. This technique permits a light anesthesia. A high level of oxygen is maintained throughout the surgery, which promotes safety. Local anesthesia is preferred by some patients and is completely adequate for this purpose. General anesthesia requires the services of an expert anesthesiologist, who charges separately. His fee is explained in the preoperative instructions. If you have a local or general anesthesia, in either case there will be no pain during the operation.

(5) How long is the operation?

The actual surgical time may vary, depending on the amount of surgery necessary for each patient. A face lift usually requires about two hours and eyelid surgery one hour.

(6) How long is the hospital stay?

The usual hospital stay is three days. Admission is usually one day prior to the operation at about 11:00 A.M. and discharge time is about 10:00 A.M. the second or third day after surgery. Admission to the hospital may seem unnecessarily early, but is necessary in order to perform the required laboratory work and examinations by the resident surgeon and anesthesiologist. Although the room accommodations are booked well in advance of admission, it may not always be possible to have the accommodation you desire on admission to the hospital. Every attempt on my part will be made to handle this problem to your advantage.

(7) Are bandages applied?

Bandages are applied to the head and neck after a face lift. These are removed 48 hours after surgery. Bandages may or may not be applied to the eyelids for a few hours. Following removal of the bandages, ice compresses are applied to the eyes for several hours. Although this will not prevent all bruising and swelling it will help minimize it. After leaving the hospital, the use of these ice compresses may be continued at home from time to time, if you find them comfortable. Bandages are applied for several reasons, one being to keep the operated area as immobile as possible, therefore it is also important that telephone calls and visitors should be kept to a minimum for the first 48 hours after the operation. But postoperative pain is rare; and whatever discomfort there may be is usually mild, short-lived and is easily handled with routine medication.

(8) *When are the stitches removed?*

Most eyelid stitches will be removed on the second day after the operation. The remainder are removed on the third or fourth day. Some stitches in front of the ears are removed on the sixth or seventh day after a face lift. In most instances, all remaining stitches are removed by the tenth day. Removing stitches is quick and uncomplicated. But you must remain in the New York area for a minimum of 10 days following facial surgery and one week following eyelid surgery so that the removal may be done. *Stitches are always removed by my nurses.*

(9) *When can make-up be applied?*

Eye make-up may usually be applied five days following the removal of the last sutures. This includes mascara, eye shadow and artificial eyelashes. Facial make-up can usually be applied about the tenth day. At this time, you may have to use some type of covering cream if there are still bruises below the eyes. It is important to remove all make-up very thoroughly, using an upward motion, at the end of the day. Oiled eye pads are recommended for the removal of eye make-up. My office staff will provide detailed instructions on make-up during the postoperative period.

(10) *When may I get my hair done?*

On the fourth day following surgery, you may comb your hair out by using a solution of warm water and a large toothed comb. Your first shampoo will not be possible until the eighth day following surgery. You may do this yourself or go to a hairdresser who is acquainted with the special procedure of the first hairset after plastic surgery. My office can recommend someone suitable. Rollers may be used but loosely. A hair dryer may also be used but at the "comfort zone" (never hot), since at this time you may not have full sensation in the areas operated upon. Tinting and coloring usually may be done about three weeks following the operation.

(11) Is the hair shaved in preparation for the operation?

The hair is not shaved. At the time of surgery, a small margin of hair behind the ears is trimmed where the incision will be. A similar area is trimmed inside the hairline above the ears. Neither area is visible once the hair is combed over the incision.

(12) Who takes care of me after surgery?

Except on Fridays and the weekends, you will be visited every day in the hospital by me. If for unforeseen reasons, I am unable to visit you, you will be seen by one of my staff. There is an expert team of associates and assistants always in attendance, who are continuously in touch with me. It is also not possible for me to visit you the night of admission to the hospital. Therefore, it is important that any unresolved questions be discussed prior to admission, if necessary, by a further visit to the office.

(13) Who actually performs the operation?

I PERFORM ALL SURGERY ON MY PATIENTS. I do have assistants who play an active role in your operation by assisting me just as the anesthetist and nurse do. However, the actual operative procedure is performed by me.

(14) What happens in the postoperative period?

You must remember that before you see the improvement you are expecting you will go through a standard postoperative period in which you will look quite battered and bruised followed by another temporary period of time when you may look "strange" to yourself. This varies considerably with each individual. When both facial and eyelid surgery is performed together you should set aside three weeks for recovery. At the end of this time most patients are able to appear in public although the scars may need camouflaging with make-up. In some patients this time may be shortened by a few days and in others a slightly longer period is required. I think you should also bear in mind that in some patients undergoing facial and eyelid surgery, there is a temporary period of slight emotional depression immediately following the surgery, during the period of time when you look your worst. This is quite normal and should not alarm you. It is not easy to look bruised and swollen, particularly when natural expectations are towards improving your appearance. Fortunately this period usually passes rather quickly.

(15) Are private nurses available?

Although not a necessity, some patients feel happier knowing that someone will be with them following surgery. Some hospitals require the patient to book private nurses at the time of admission. At other hospitals we are able to arrange for nurses in advance. In spite of booking well in advance of surgery, there is no guarantee that nurses will be available because of the critical shortage of such help.

If you have any other questions be sure to get them answered in advance by me or my office. Many members of my office staff have been with me for years and are thoroughly informed, trained and able to answer questions that may occur to you. Well meaning friends are not a good source of information. Find out everything you want to know. A well informed patient is a happy one.

19

"Hello, Room Service? I'm the Rhinoplasty in 310"

This was the title of a paper written by an eminently qualified plastic surgeon in New York, Dr. J. Douglas Lake, a dissident who got fed up with conditions in New York City hospitals and opened an in-and-out surgical suite at a hotel.

The paper was published in the magazine *Medical Economics* in March 1976 and is reprinted here by special permission of the publisher and Dr. Lake, who gave me my copy with his personal notation, "This can save a patient $1,000 to $4,000 and give better care."

As he tells it . . .

One evening as I settled myself comfortably at home with a Jack Daniels to watch "Hawaii Five-O," my phone rang. The near-hysterical mother of a hospitalized girl on whom I'd performed a rhinoplasty that day told me her daughter had been bleeding for over an hour; she couldn't get the floor nurses to take any corrective action. I phoned the hospital and went through two nurses who spoke what sounded like a Far-Eastern tongue. Neither could give me a comprehensible report or understand instructions in English. Finally I was able to communicate successfully—in Spanish—with the night supervisor and get the bleeding stopped.

That was the last straw. In 25 years of practice in New York City, I'd become increasingly unhappy with the general hospitals here. While the city has plenty of hospital beds, the relatively few you'd want to put a member of your family into are jealously guarded by doctors who got there first. Delays of four to six weeks before nonemergency surgery are common in my experience, and conditions and attitudes in the O.R. (Operating Room) are often far from ideal—particularly for patients undergoing cosmetic surgery, which O.R. personnel tend to regard as frivolous. In one hospital, all surgery performed under local anesthesia must be scheduled after 1 P.M.—but the O.R. staff goes off duty at 3. A surgeon sometimes finds himself working alone in the middle of a major procedure.

Post-op care for cosmetic surgery patients ranges from benign neglect to flat failure to carry out instructions, with the surgeon, of course, ultimately held accountable. And for all of this, the hospitals are demanding $150 to $250 a day for rooms that are often small, dingy, and unkempt—with up to $1,000 in preadmission deposits from cosmetic surgery patients, since their insurance may not cover the procedure.

The bleeding incident epitomized my constant struggle to provide suitable accommodations and effective team care for my patients. And with my practice volume rising sharply and my nerves fraying, I knew I had to find a better way to meet the medical, psychological, and economic needs of my patients.

Clearly the answer lay in some form of private in-and-out surgery. Then I remembered that an old friend, now retired from medicine, had maintained an office in a midtown hotel and occasionally did plastic surgical procedures there, keeping the patient overnight. Why not an in-and-out surgical hotel suite?

The location I chose was in the relatively crime-free upper East Side. Several hotels were not receptive to my idea, but the Hotel Westbury, one of New York's elegant residential hotels, was most responsive. The management offered me a light, airy, and thoroughly attractive upper-floor suite, consisting of a sitting room, two bedrooms, a bath, and a kitchenette. I could immediately see the sitting room and the interior bedroom and bath as operating, sterilization, and scrub rooms.

Only the O.R. needed any considerable alterations—such as conversion of the bathroom sink into a scrub sink and the shower into a sterilizer alcove, as well as the installation of operating lights. Disposable drapes and utensils and miniaturized electronic equipment made the rest of the job easy. My resuscitation kit, for instance, fits in a case no larger than a small suitcase.

I arranged for preoperative screening to be done by a local laboratory. And, to avoid any conflict with state and municipal ordinances governing hospitals and clinics, I didn't set up any recovery room. Instead, patients who may require postoperative care check into a hotel room adjacent to my suite between 10 and 11 A.M., preparatory to my normal 1 P.M. operating time.

They are sedated and brought to the operating room by wheelchair. In the O.R. I administer a quick-acting general anesthetic, establish the appropriate local anesthesia, and, with the patient again conscious, proceed with the operation. Afterward he's returned to his hotel room and remains there under sedation for the night. One of my nurses makes frequent checks on patients throughout the night and can be summoned immediately by a buzzer system. In most cases a patient leaves the hotel the next day.

The fact that the patient checks into the hotel himself not only avoids conflict with health ordinances but obviates the need for me to maintain expensive floor space. I have as many rooms at my disposal for patients as are vacant in the hotel. My staff of five nurses, some of whom hold other employment, too, are also used only as needed. On days when there is no surgery, my office staff consists of one highly competent secretary.

Since we do only cosmetic surgery, the nurses are oriented toward those procedures and patients. The teamwork and nursing service are far beyond what you'll find in most general hospitals. If the patient desires, a private-duty nurse can also be hired through a neighborhood registry.

Since May, 1974, we've performed hundreds of procedures, covering the whole range of cosmetic surgery from blepharoplasty to breast implants, with not one untoward occurrence, much less an emergency postoperative complication.

Only four patients were admitted to a hospital instead during this period, three for procedures that were postoperatively unstable and one because of an old, quiescent coronary condition that his internist wanted to monitor.

From both a medical and an economic standpoint this system has proven ideal for my patients and myself. Operations are scheduled without the long delays that can be stressful in themselves. The patient spends a postoperative period—never longer than is actually required—in the comfort and privacy of a fine hotel, with fully responsive nursing care. Linen and kitchen services are at his command in surroundings that none but the most expensive hospitals can match for luxury and privacy. Parents and relatives can check in with the patient, easing their anxiety and eliminating the inconvenience of traveling to and from a hospital.

While my patients are enjoying these benefits, they are also saving hundreds of dollars in hospital costs. The average hospital stay for my cosmetic surgery patients was three days; in most cases they're now home in one day. I've seen a hospital bill for a blepharoplasty that totaled

$3,500; the same patient would have paid $50 to $75 at the Westbury. One of my patients paid her first-class, round-trip air fare for a vacation in England with the money she'd saved on hospitalization.

Most insurance carriers, in cases that fall within their range of coverage, deal with my "hotelized" patients just as they would if they were hospitalized as inpatients. The use of a hotel rather than a hospital saves them considerable money, too.

True, my hotel suite costs more in rent than an ordinary office would. But this better way of practice more than pays for itself in increased productivity, enhanced patient relationships, and vastly improved working conditions.

Since this paper was written, Dr. Lake has changed his location to a suite in the Hotel Alrae, which is as well equipped, well kept, as posh and beautifully appointed as any private clinic I have seen anywhere—and certainly more inviting than any hospital I've ever seen, and I've been in and out of a lot of them all over the world with a diabetic husband who has required frequent hospitalization. I mention this only to let you know that I do have perhaps a better-than-average basis for comparison of hospitals and while I have nothing against them—in fact we've had excellent service in most of them—I personally would not consider having my facelift done in a general hospital, for the very reasons mentioned by most of the qualified plastic surgeons I've talked to.

In fact the last two times I've had to rush my husband to the hospital's emergency room, there were emergency patients lined up in the hallway ahead of him waiting for a room to become available. Each time he had to share a semi-private room (no private ones available) with another patient who was seriously ill.

Certainly under conditions like this, a cosmetic surgery patient couldn't help but be regarded with resentment. Many doctors have told me they've had cosmetic surgery patients who were either ignored or mistreated by the hospital staff whose attitude is that such patients are only in on an "ego trip."

One doctor said, "I'd fire any nurse I caught mistreating a patient, but trying to catch them is the problem."

Dr. Lake would like to see more plastic surgeons operate outside hospitals not only to help cut down the enormous costs of hospital stays but to bring the option of cosmetic surgery to a larger public.

I'm sure many more would opt for it if they could have it done in a setup like his—a hospital operating room in a hotel. And with room service yet!

When his patients check in at the "hospital" where he operates, they are technically changing their residence. When he walks down the hall to their hotel room to make a call, he is therefore making what constitutes a "house call." How many doctors make house calls anymore?

He is so enthusiastic about his procedure that he invited me into his operating room to watch him perform an upper blepharoplasty (operation on upper eyelids) on a sixty-eight-year-old woman, the mother of a well-known Broadway musical director.

The operating room itself is an exact prototype of a hospital OR, impeccably, glisteningly immaculate and sterile; very top drawer, beyond reproach compared with all the hospital operating rooms I have seen.

The reception room of Dr. Lake's hotel-hospital is far more inviting than run-of-the-mill hospital reception rooms, with luscious thick carpeting, attractive and comfortable chairs, a pleasing decor.

Dr. Lake, a tall, vigorous, outdoorsman type, exudes a feeling of warmth, rapport, and professionalism with his patients. He gave the patient, Anna, a pill before preparing her for the operation. (I was dressed in a disposable paper gown, mask, and cap, covering all my hair, for my observation of the procedure.) Then he gave her an injection of Brevital, a quick-acting pain-killer that knocks the patient out for only a few minutes; thus no problem with the larynx, no memory of pain, no stimulation of adrenalin, and no ensuing potential of bleeding. It is frequently described as a "sub-general anesthetic."

During the brief knockout, the doctor was able to insert the Novocain needles in the eye area with no discomfort to the patient.

The operation itself was performed while the patient was able to respond to questions from the doctor. She obediently remained quiet when he requested but loquaciously proclaimed her great love for the doctor and gave forth with "family secrets" that might have come straight out of a soap opera.

Following the operation, Dr. Lake invited me to question the patient, who said, "I feel fine. There is no pain or discomfort. There never has been, even when he operated on me last year for my facelift."

Although it was not necessary, she checked into a room in the hotel for an extra night and a friend stayed with her.

In general, Dr. Lake feels that too much emphasis is placed on a physician's affiliations with hospitals and specialty boards.

"The best plastic surgeons do not work in the biggest hospitals," he told me, "because the big hospitals do not give them facilities. I'm speaking of *cosmetic* plastic surgeons. For instance, there is a man here in New York who does very fine nose jobs, and he works in a tiny out-of-the-way hospital that is very decrepit. But he works there because they let him do five or six rhinoplasties a day, which is what his practice calls for. He is on the staff of one of our big teaching institutions. He never goes near the place because if he does, they want him to work in clinics where he can do maybe only two or three operations a week.

"Hospital appointments are often largely political. And cosmetic surgery generally does not require the facilities of a big institution. I'm not speaking of large plastic reconstructive work. If what you want is a facelift, I'd say you should be suspicious of a man who makes too much of his hospital connections. He may be using that to compensate for his own lack of ability. In effect what he's saying is, 'I work at mid-city *teaching* hospital and my competitor who works at mid-city *municipal* hospital obviously can't be as good.' This is not true. Those things are usually political and they are traps."

In his opinion the medical specialty boards are also traps, whether it's the Board of Plastic Surgery, Internal Medicine, Ophthamology, Cardiology—whatever.

"These are all boards organized under the auspices of the AMA, created to review the doctor's training, set up standards, give examinations, and award diplomas certifying that he has a certain basic competence," he explained. "But they do not attest that he is a *good* doctor, and that is very important. All they're saying is that you're going to get average competent care—but it doesn't mean that you're going to get super care.

"In cosmetic surgery everyone wants superb care. In my opinion there is no such thing as a *fair* result in cosmetic surgery. Results are either excellent or unsatisfactory. A woman does not have her eyelids done to look a little better. She either wants them to look very good or it's not worth the trouble."

So how would *he* go about finding a facelifter who is really good?

"There are men in this country who have very little formal training but who do superb work," he replied. "This man in New York who does nothing but noses has had very little formal training but he turns out beautiful noses one after the other like sausages. I had a friend in Los Angeles—he's now dead—who did nothing but facelifts. He did beautiful facelifts. All he did was facelifts.

"Plastic surgery is not a very intellectual specialty such as, say, pediatrics, neurology, or neurosurgery. It's an *artistic* specialty, it's an art form, it's in the fingers. In our specialty we have notorious cases of men who write textbooks, who lecture widely, who hold national positions, but who are *terrible* operators. They do awful work. Their textbooks contain nonsense. We have others who have never written textbooks, who perhaps in their entire life have only published one paper but they are absolute masters in cosmetic operations. The only thing you can compare it with is musical ability. One person can study musical theory at Juilliard for five years and still not be a good pianist; then there's the boy who comes down from the hills and with only a little training can play beautifully."

A surgeon's background is an indicator of whether he is equipped to take care of you competently, he said, but beyond that you should look at the *results,* talk to his former patients who have had facelifts.

Many of course do not want to discuss their facelifts with anyone, although in my experience I have found the majority of people most co-operative in talking confidentially when they could be helpful—either to me in the preparation of this book or to others seeking information about what the operation entails and advice on how to choose a doctor.

Says Dr. Lake, "Every surgeon should be able to arrange for interviews with some of his patients—those who've had a facelift, a nose job, a chin reduction—who are willing to say, 'Here's what I went through and here's how I look.' Of course there's always the risk of a second-rate doctor showing off only his best specimens, never the bad ones. In talking to patients, it's best to stick with those whose doctors have had uniformly good results."

How would you know this? It's not easy to check out and I personally have my doubts that you could find an infallible facelifter. But it's worth a try. Your best bet is to follow up on all recommendations, look at the specimens, listen to the pros and cons, get second opinions, and above all, *investigate* before you *invest* in a facelift.

20

Complications
and Consolation

Even in the hands of the best-qualified doctors, a facelift is not risk-free.

What are the chances of complications, infections, or unsatisfactory results? What can be done? Is there any guarantee of success?

Your biggest risk, as you know by now, is in trying to latch on to the right doctor, not only one who is highly qualified with all the proper credentials but one who can give *you* the kind of facelift that *you* want.

As one plastic surgeon put it, "There is always a risk but the risk is not in the operation being successful but in the patient being satisfied. So I always tell my patients to be realistic; they will not look younger, they will look just fresher and more rested."

That's what they all tell you. Baloney! Anybody who's paying for a facelift these days is entitled to a little more than looking just fresher and more rested.

But then you could come out with eyes and cheeks bulging like a squirrel's.

Some doctors will tell you that your chances of dying on the operating table while having a facelift are less likely than being hit by a bus or zonked by a root canal. Others say that the *more* or *less* success of a facelift operation can be divided into four categories—poor, fair, good, and excellent.

Somewhere between these extremes of opinion lies the question most people want answers to: *What are the hazards involved in having a facelift?*

Some operations do go astray. The biggest risk, many surgeons say, is the accidental cutting of one of the branches of the facial nerve, which may leave the patient with a paralyzed forehead or drooping lip for about three to six months—but it usually can be corrected.

There is also the possibility of a hematoma, which is a swelling containing blood and must be treated; and of course there is the possibility of an infection or a reaction to drugs, which can happen in any operation.

Such "accidents" as a stroke or heart attack are no more likely to happen during a facelift than at any other time, doctors say. In fact, if you're in good health and in the hands of a good doctor, the chances of complications or infections from a facelift are minimal. Infection of the face is not common because of the rich blood supply to the face. There is always the danger of bleeding following surgery—caused by the effect of anesthesia on the blood vessels—but this is usually not serious.

As with any surgery, there is *no guarantee* of the outcome or results. As one plastic surgeon said, "You can't make guarantees when you're dealing with flesh and blood. All you can do is make a stab at statistics, like Jimmy the Greek rattling off odds; I'd say there's a 1 per cent chance—if you're going into details beyond death and disaster—of permanent nerve damage to some of the muscles in the face; a 5 to 8 per cent chance of hematoma; a 1 to 2 per cent of a bad scar . . . That's about all."

Another put it this way, "Our techniques today are pretty much standardized. We've learned what causes serious cosmetic problems and we stay away from them. If we get a result which is less than normal, it's usually because a blood clot formed or the patient didn't heal right, or some minor mishap, but usually these things can be corrected, and I'd say that in practically every case a satisfactory anatomical or physical result can be produced."

This is an understatement considering the remarkable repair work that has been done on some seriously botched-up cases turned out by the hacks.

In fact, one of the truly bright lights on the facelift horizon is that if you wind up with a bad job on the first round, you *can* have it fixed. This should be some consolation, though remember—it's better to have it done right in the first place.

LIFT TIPS:

Q & A

21

The Questions People Ask

Many of the questions you've always wanted to ask about facelifts have already been answered. Many others remain in my Q & A files compiled through the years. I think they cover just about everything you could possibly think of to ask. Some people do ask the darndest things! Like, what if a facelift doesn't "take"?

Here are the questions—and answers—based on interviews with scores of doctors and hundreds of patients, as well as my years of research and examination of the medical literature on the subject.

The answers have been sifted, sorted, and culled with thoughtful care and my best judgment, in the most jumbled mess of contradictions, controversy, professional conspiracy, and confusion I ever got into. I pity the poor souls who start out on their own trying to get a straight answer from the professionals. Fortunately, I have had the time and resources that few people have to pursue the answers—and thus give *you* some shortcuts to making what could be one of the most important decisions of your life.

Keep in mind—for every answer you get here, you can find an "expert" on practically every street corner to dispute it. But remember—*Caveat emptor!*

Does it hurt?

This is usually the first and most common question women ask. Is the facelift painful or isn't it? There is no categorical answer to this one because each person reacts differently. Personally, I've been amazed at the number of patients—by far the majority—who've told me they had absolutely no pain at all. Some doctors tend to minimize the possibility of pain in order to sell the operation. Most, if they're honest, will tell you there is always some pain and discomfort in any surgical procedure; but it's more painful for some than for others. Some say the rhinoplasty (nose operation) is the most painful; others say it's the least painful. One woman told me hers was "excruciating." The majority say there is some discomfort but no pain. The eyelid operation probably has minimal discomfort. The facelift operation usually leaves you black and blue for a few days, and it stands to reason that you'll feel at least slight discomfort. Some patients also experience a numbness of the earlobes or cheek, or neuralgic pains behind the ears, which may last for several months and be very bothersome. One woman said that after her anesthetic wore off, "my scalp ached and I felt like a balloon." Many say it's not half as bad as going to the dentist. And even those who felt pain will usually tell you, "It's like having a baby. You're so happy that you forget the pain."

Will my face look like a mask?

This is usually the second question women ask. Most doctors will tell you no. But there are an awful lot of mask-faces in Palm Springs. It depends on how much you want done and how often you've had it done. Those with the most mask-like faces usually have had several lifts and/or really prefer the tighter face to make them look twenty years younger. And you can always find doctors to oblige.

But a facelift doesn't inevitably look like a mask, as many people assume, and most of them don't. Naturally, your facial expression is altered somewhat by the pulled-back skin widening the eyes, but there are many qualified and skilled doctors who know how to do a facelift without pulling you too tight, changing your expression too much, or leaving you with that slit-in-the face non-smile. One of my friends in Palm Springs, with one of the prettiest smiles I know, recently had a facelift in Beverly Hills and came back with her lovely smile and facial expressions still intact—quite a contrast to the masks so prevalent here. Her doctor doesn't believe in making patients look too much younger—ten years at the most—and simply refuses to give them tighter lifts even if they insist on it. Most competent and conscientious plastic surgeons prefer *not* to do a lift that changes the face too drastically. So, whether you'll look like a mask or not is mostly up to *you*. You certainly don't have to.

Will there be scars? Will they be visible?

There is always a scar in any kind of surgery. Wherever a cut is made, there will be a scar. But the art of the plastic surgeon is in placing these scars in natural lines and creases so they will not be obvious after the healing process has been completed. Also the fine techniques and materials used for repairing the scars have a lot to do with the final look of a scar. Patients must understand that there is a normal maturation process for a scar and this may take several weeks or months. A scar that is red and slightly raised a few days after surgery, may be practically invisible in a few months.

I must say that one of the things that has impressed me most about plastic surgery in general is the vast improvement in techniques to deal with scars. This is obvious when comparing facelifts done twenty and twenty-five years ago and those being done today. I have friends who came out of those earlier facelifts looking rather dreadful. Some of them have scars that still show if you know where to look, or areas around the eyes, chin, or neck that are still conspicuously too tight, or pulled the wrong way. By contrast, among those I have examined recently, close up and some even in bright sunlight and without makeup, it is often nearly impossible for me to see the fresh, new scars on their eyelids, behind their ears, under the chin— even when they point them out. And I have good eyesight.

Is it true that only your hairdresser will know?

No. He or she may be the first to know but not the only one. Your best friends will know, even if you don't tell them. So will casual acquaintances and even strangers if they're snoopily sniffing out who has or has not had a facelift, which is a favorite pastime in some circles.

Will your husband or lover know? Is there any way for them not to know?

Not unless they're blind. But if they really love you, it shouldn't matter. (I told you—some people ask the darndest things.)

Is it better to tell—or not to tell—your husband and friends and family?

Surprisingly, many women who should know better are still plagued by this dilemma. Whether you choose to tell them is your business but you should know up front that they're going to know anyway and will be buzzing behind your back— unless you got ripped off with a facelift that didn't do a thing for you. If you only came out looking "fresh and rested," they can guess you had one; and if you got enough of a lift to make the difference you probably want, they'll know for sure. Personally, I'm for bringing it out of the closet but maybe that's because I live in California. If more people would admit it, the others wouldn't feel so guilt-ridden.

If you prefer not to tell, what can you do if someone pointedly asks if you've had your face done?

You can either lie, tell the clods it's none of their damn business, or do what I would do—smile (if you're still able to), and say, "Sure, how do you like it?" Then be prepared for anything. The silliest thing is to play dumb and pretend you don't know what in heaven's name they're talking about or why everybody is staring at you, especially if you're seventyish and suddenly pop out with a twenty-five- or thirty-year-old face.

What should you say to someone you know who has just had a facelift and admits it?

This too can be sticky. If you say, "You look much younger," she could take offense because you're implying she looked old before. If you don't say anything, it could be worse because she has spent a lot of money and gone to a lot of trouble hoping for a noticeable change, and if nobody notices, it would all be for nothing. Follow Dear Abby's advice and just say, "You look great!" That will cover everything.

What about bandages? How long do they stay on?

A lot of people think they're going to look like mummies for a while. That was true years ago. No more. Most doctors have decided that bandages are ineffectual, inconvenient, uncomfortable, and unnecessary. Now, usually the day after their facelifts, patients can shampoo their hair, fluff it out, put on a kerchief and dark glasses—and off they go.

Shouldn't you stay in bed or at least take it easy and rest for the first few days after a facelift?

Most doctors advise this. Some patients do, some don't. A friend of mine with a history of high blood pressure obeyed doctor's orders and stayed in bed a few days. Her boyfriend was annoyed. "It's ridiculous," he said. "I had my face done this morning, I've been swimming already, and I'm playing in a bridge tournament this afternoon." He wasn't even black and blue. He was gorgeous, as always. But then he hadn't had a full facelift that day—just a few little tucks. His eye and chin crinkles are nipped as regularly as most women pluck their eyebrows. On second thought, probably more so.

What must I do to get in shape for this?

Another common question from facelift candidates. Doctors advise you to avoid drugs of all sorts—aspirin particularly, because it inhibits blood clotting. *It is extremely important to advise your doctor of any medications you're taking.* Also, most doctors advise you to give up alcohol and tobacco for at least a couple of weeks. And if you're overweight, they'll tell you to lose weight before your operation for better results. Again, not all doctors or all patients follow these rules. There are no Gallup-Poll-type statistics to back me up, but in my personal case-history notebooks it's usually an *overweight woman* who has the stroke or heart attack during a facelift. Naturally, this doesn't mean all overweight women are going to have strokes on the operating table. One woman told me she just took her Valium and three martinis and woke up looking beautiful. The miracle is that so many turn out as well as they do.

How and when do I know if I really need a facelift?

Probably when you look in the mirror and can't stand what you see, though a great many women, and men too—men especially—have their first little tuck when they glimpse their first little wrinkle.

How long does a facelift last?

This is one of the most common questions and subject to the most variable answers, myths, and misconceptions. It depends on many factors: your *age* when you have it done, *how much* of a lift you have, i.e., a few tucks, a "mini-lift" or full facelift; *how many* and *what kind* of lifts you've had, i.e., chemical peels or plastic surgery; your hereditary characteristics such as bone structure and type of skin; and your general lifestyle—eating and drinking habits, exposure to the sun, emotional problems.

Personally, I'm surprised at the number of otherwise intelligent people I meet *who think a facelift should last forever.* Of course it doesn't. Why should it? Does your car last forever? When it wears out, you buy a new one. Most people don't wait for it to wear out. It's the same with facelifts.

When properly done at the right age by the right doctor a good facelift should last you at least eight to ten years; I've seen many that have lasted much longer and many that had to be redone in six months. It's the choice of the doctor that makes the difference.

What is the best age to have a facelift—for the best results?

Most doctors agree that the best age is in your forties. Some say they won't do a facelift on anyone under forty. I've never personally met any of these doctors. My general impression is that you'll have no problem finding a doctor to lift you wherever you want it, no matter how young or old you are. Jolie Gabor has just had her latest lifts—full facelift, eyelift, full facial chemical peel *ALL AT THE SAME TIME*. At age eighty-nine yet! A real optimist . . .

How many facelifts can you have?

Some people have as many as three or four over a period of twenty years or so. Some have frequent nips and tucks in between. It depends on how young you want to continue looking for how long—and probably on how many trips to the lifter you can afford.

Does a facelift include the eyelids too, or are they separate operations?

Again, this depends on the doctor and on whether you need both face and eyes done. The standard facelift removes sagging skin and jowls, tightening the areas around the cheeks, chin, neck, and the temples. It does not eliminate deep frown lines or "smile" wrinkles. The eyelid operation, the most popular form of cosmetic surgery, removes pouches and lines from under the eye and the droopy, baggy excess skin on the upper eyelids. Some doctors perform both the face- and eyelifts at the same time; others do them in separate operations.

Should people who get bags under their eyes in their twenties have them removed then or wait?

"That's an ideal time to operate. I've done many at that age," says a top New York plastic surgeon. Bags under the eyes at an early age are almost always inherited.

What if a facelift doesn't "take"?

I'm frankly puzzled by this question. A facelift doesn't "take" or not "take." It doesn't just suddenly "drop" overnight. The sags and bags have been taken out, removed, they're gone—into the doctor's trash bag. They don't jump out and come back the next day. Whether your sags and wrinkles have been sheared off by the knife or the peel, what's done is done, some of your skin is gone, there's no question of a facelift "taking." It's more a question of what *you* expected, and how much the doctor took off—too much or too little—and whether he botched up your face or only gave you a "mini-lift" that might not last a year or six months.

What is a "mini-lift"? Does it work?

There are a lot of questions and talk about "mini-lifts." Doctors generally don't like that term because basically a "mini-lift" is what you get in a sham operation performed by schlocks who hawk their wares as a full facelift (see Chapter 17). Ethical doctors will tell you whether you need a full facelift or a partial one, only a little work—skin tightening, nips and tucks in certain areas. If you prefer to call this a "mini-lift," go ahead.

Are there "mini-hospitals" where patients can go during recovery, rather than to their homes?

A great number of recuperation hideaways—halfway houses for people recovering from cosmetic surgery—have sprung up in the Los Angeles area, and they have already created problems for health authorities. They are not licensed as nursing or convalescent homes. They are usually staffed by nurse's aides or lay attendants who do everything from preparing meals, removing bandages, and driving patients to and from the doctor's office to watching for complications. One patient was rushed to the hospital in a diabetic coma. (She probably didn't tell her doctor she was a diabetic.) The average length of stay in these hostelries—often the private homes of nurses or attendants who work in plastic surgeons' offices—is only two or three days.

One strong point of agreement among doctors from coast

to coast is that a facelift doesn't require more than a two- or three-day recovery period for the "normal" or average person in good health. Many doctors only keep patients overnight and send them home the next day—or to a hotel, motel, condominium, a recovery ranch, or private "villa" (as in Palm Springs) until they feel ready to face the public again. Most doctors also advise that you have a friend, a companion, a member of your family, or a private nurse, if you want to hire one, with you for the first few days; this service isn't provided in your facelift fee. Personally I've seen enough minor mishaps in this early post-operative period to convince me that an on-duty doctor's attendant is more essential than deluxe surroundings. Naturally I'd prefer both, wouldn't you?

Do doctors use silicone in facelifts?
Not anymore.

Does a facelift guarantee beauty?
Are you kidding?

Does it guarantee anything?
No.

Can you be made to look like anyone you want?
Try Elvis Presley, not Elizabeth Taylor.

Is it better to have it done in the winter or summer?
Any time, any clime.

How many years can you expect it to take off your age?
An average of between eight and ten—much more if you take your sweet-girl-graduate picture to an operator who's willing to transpose the face on a dowager's hump. Some can. But don't ask me to tell you who they are.

Does the doctor make a sketch of how you will look?
Sometimes, yes—with $$$$$ signs beside each section of your face. That's the time for you to split. Fast.

Are your motivations important? Does this in any way affect the doctor's decision to do a facelift?
For my answer to this I suggest that you turn back and re-

view Chapter 6—Darling, I'm Dripping . . . I Want a Facelift from the Ankles Up . . . I'll repeat here, for emphasis, that in my opinion all those pious admonishments about your "motivations"—and the medical literature is crammed with them— are utter hogwash. Better you should look into the motivations of the cosmetic surgeons. Since when are they mind doctors? Typical is this warning, "The main reason cosmetic surgery must be approached with caution is that it is so tricky a matter psychologically." It could be your surgeon needs a shrink. Check it out. . . . In one medical Q & A appears the following:

Q *My husband wants me to have plastic surgery—is that a good enough reason?*

A No, all doctors agree that this is a poor reason. It should be something you have done because you want it.

I don't believe it. I think it was a made up Q & A. First, if your husband thinks you need a facelift, you'd better darn well run, don't walk, to your nearest qualified facelifter. Second, if all doctors agree that this is a poor reason, they all need their own heads examined. Third, I have yet to meet a woman who had her face done because her husband or anyone else told her she needed it or pressured her into it.

Doctors make a big to-do about "motivations," "social pressures," and "outside forces" heaving you into a facelift.

The nitty-gritty of it is, the MDs don't give the rest of the human race credit for having any modicum of common, ordinary horse sense.

Most people are bright enough to know why they want a facelift. Most people have it done to please themselves, not any "outside forces."

If you want a facelift to hold a husband or a lover or a job, that's *your* business, not the plastic surgeon's. It's his job to fix your face, not your psyche.

22

The Trouble with Noses

Apparently a lot of people are paranoid about their noses and this can cause problems. Your nose occupies the most prominent spot in your face. It sits there hogging all the attention; and if it's a bumped, humped, curved, beaked, bulbous, or big nose, I suppose it could be a dreadful curse if you can't learn to live with it.

If it bothers you, it would seem to me that the simple solution would be to have a nose job and get it over with, as many thousands have done. For years the rhinoplasty was the most popular form of cosmetic surgery and still is one of the most popular, exceeded only by the blepharoplasty (eyelids).

I've known literally hundreds of people who've had nose jobs—many of them my own friends and relatives—and I've never known any of them to make a big deal of it psychologically, either before or after the operation.

They didn't like their noses, so they had them altered. Simple as that.

But the top, most reputable plastic surgeons agree that it isn't quite that simple because many people have developed a fixation about that bump on their nose, many others have preconceived notions about the kind of nose they want, and it might not fit their face, and many are not well enough informed about what to expect in the post-operative period.

Some plastic surgeons feel that rhinoplasty is the most difficult and exacting of cosmetic operations, not because of the operation itself, which is relatively simple, but because designing the right kind of nose requires a lot of work with the patient.

"The aim of the plastic surgeon is to make the nose fit the face, and in fact the entire body image of the patient," one doctor explained. "If a young lady comes in, and she's really a kind of Betty Co-ed, it's okay to give her a cute little button nose. But if she's more sophisticated and projects a different body image, she should have a different kind of nose."

Even doctors who do not dwell on psychological factors in a facelift generally agree that there is a greater possibility of emotional depression and other problems after nose surgery than other cosmetic operations.

They have plenty of case histories to back them up. One of the silliest of these was the dummy who had a nose job and afterward was sorry she did it because: "The truth is that I miss my old nose. I regret the fact that a part of me, a part of my heritage, has been cut away."

She must have been a great joy to her doctors. At the ripe age of seventeen she had decided that her nose was too large for her face. She spent three years weighing the pros and cons of an operation and searching for the right surgeon to do it. She didn't like the way it turned out the first time, so he did it over. It cost her 50 per cent more than she had counted on.

This made her angry. "I feel cheated, exploited, abused," she raged. Yet, she admitted later it wasn't all the plastic surgeon's fault. What really zapped her was an old photograph of her great-grandfather, hanging in the family dining room, which suddenly reminded her that the nose she had been born with, the one she had thought was too large for her face, was also her father's nose. And she still saw it every day in Grandpa's photograph. "It was one of the few real tangible links I had with my past."

At last report, the young lady, a college graduate, was hoping she'd feel better when her newest nose was unbandaged. She was looking forward to having a small, delicate, straight nose in a few months. "But at the moment," she wrote, in her mood of depression, "I wonder why, in this age of *Roots,* I was so eager to have mine destroyed. I feel abused, and I feel like a fool."

Lord knows how many nose jobs she's had by now.

Then there was the elderly woman who came into the office of a New York plastic surgeon with a really terrible rhinoplasty she'd had done many years ago, way back in the forties. As the doctor described the case to me:

"Her nose was all caved in, so with plastic implants we built it up so it looked pretty good for a woman of her age. She's quite an old lady. And for about four to six weeks afterward she was ecstatic, she was in heaven with her new nose.

"She looked better, she was fine. Then she began this— well, it wasn't right, she wasn't happy. About a month or so later she started saying she was *very* unhappy, *very* depressed, she was going to commit suicide. I did another minor revision on her nose and again she went from being overelated to overdepressed. I sent her to another doctor, a top plastic surgeon and professor in a leading New York medical center. From him, she went on to someone else, and then someone else. No matter who did what to her, she always came out with this tremendous elation followed by a severe depression. In a situation of this kind, the operation will always fail regardless of what you do physically."

Such extreme cases are rare. But many less severe problems can be eliminated if patients are prepared, if they know exactly what a "nose job" entails and why there is—or may be —a temporary period of emotional depression following surgery. New York's famous Dr. Thomas D. Rees always gives his patients a thorough rundown of facts about cosmetic nose surgery so they will know what to expect.

Here is a summary:

• Results are more predictable in some patients than others, depending on thickness and shape of bones and cartilage, the shape of the face, heredity, age, and the thickness and condition of the skin. Thick skin precludes a delicate nasal tip.

• No two noses are the same; therefore the results of nasal surgery are never exactly the same.

• The nose is one of the main balancing features of the face and sometimes the alteration of the size and shape of the nose should also be accompanied by appropriate changes in other facial structures to obtain the best results. The chin is often augmented or altered along with the nose, particularly if it is recessed or small in size.

• The most common complication is nosebleed after surgery; this can be troublesome but is rarely serious.

• There are no external scars. Nasal plastic surgery is accomplished through incisions inside the nose which are not visible.

• The actual operating time may vary but usually requires thirty to sixty minutes; a chin implant, if required, adds fifteen to twenty minutes to that time. The usual hospital stay is three days.

• *A cast or splint is applied over your nose and remains for approximately one week* (italics mine). Light packs may or may not be inserted in your nostrils. The splints are to protect your new nose and hold down swelling.

• *In the post-operative period you will look quite battered and bruised; this is followed by another temporary period of time when you may look strange to yourself.* This varies considerably with each individual but most patients are quite presentable ten days after surgery when they can go back to school or work. In some patients a slightly longer period is required.

• In some patients undergoing nose surgery *there is a temporary period of slight emotional depression immediately following the surgery, during the period of time when you look your worst. This is quite normal and should not alarm you. It is not easy to look bruised and swollen, particularly when natural expectations are toward improving your appearance. Fortunately this period usually passes rather quickly. Do not scrutinize your nose under the splint too closely. Remember that it is swollen and taped in a high position so that it may appear too short; however, after the bandages are removed, the nose will "drop" slightly. During the first ten-day period your eyelids, cheeks, and upper lip may be swollen. The chin, too, particularly if an implant was inserted.*

• Many months are required for the final subtle changes in the nose to appear; *so be patient.*

These explicit nose-operation details from Dr. Rees are enough to give you an idea of what to expect following a rhinoplasty. There is little real physical pain or discomfort throughout the entire procedure, though it may be a big pain in the neck—or to your psyche—to wear the nose splint.

And if there's the remotest chance that you're going to miss your old nose, then skip the rhinoplasty, because you can't grow it back the way it was. The dum-dum whose "roots" were cut away with her nose bob should have thought about that ahead of time.

23

History ... Terminology ... Costs

What actually is cosmetic surgery? Is it the same as plastic surgery? If not, what is the difference?

The public generally has a limited conception of the purpose and capabilities of plastic surgery, and of its origins.

Hollywood has been so much a part of the PR hype on facelifts that a lot of people think they originated there; or that plastic surgery is a product Made in France and Sold in Hollywood, so to speak.

Modern *reconstructive* plastic surgery began as an effort to repair some of the World War I wounded. By World War II, there were more surgeons trained in plastic surgery—in this context plastic means "molding or reshaping tissues"—and using better anesthesia and improved surgical tools. As they developed more ingenious ways of reconstructing damaged parts and features, they discovered that many of the techniques used in reconstruction of the wounded could also help people look better or younger.

In the early post-war period, more and more movie stars

began having their features remolded to retain their youth and beauty, and the term aesthetic or cosmetic surgery came into use to distinguish the vanity operations from the more serious kinds of reconstructive surgery. One is a necessity, the other a luxury.

As one leading plastic surgeon who specializes in both reconstructive and cosmetic surgery explained it to me:

"In reconstructive surgery we're trying to return the patient to normal; in cosmetic surgery we're trying to surpass the normal. Both have their place but the margin for error is finer in cosmetic surgery because we're tampering with nature. I am frankly more interested in getting a person who is a recluse because of a cleft palate, for instance, back to normal than I am in a woman who wants all her friends to tell her how much better she looks after her trip to Florida."

In the early years of cosmetic surgery in this country, the cosmetic surgeons were generally derided by their peers in plastic reconstructive surgery. So strong was the feeling against them that they were often lumped in a category with abortionists.

This seems odd considering the fact that *aesthetic* or *cosmetic* surgery, as a branch of plastic surgery, actually dates back for centuries. Apparently from time immemorial people have been concerned about their facial features, and especially their noses, which were sometimes partially chopped off as punishment for adultery or frequently damaged in sword fights, and then had to be restored.

Sixteenth-century nose jobs were performed by using a skin graft from the forearm. For the graft to take on the new nose, the patient had to keep his arm planted against his nose for nearly a month.

According to Chicago's Dr. Peter McKinney, from the earliest origins of plastic surgery techniques, some of which predate 1000 B.C. its foremost objectives have remained the same—the removal or improvement of disfiguring pathological conditions and the restoration of normal appearance. Following is his brief history of plastic surgery:

As a specialty, plastic surgery is fairly young, and important advances have been made largely in response to the bodily damage wrought by major wars of the 20th century. The adjective "plastic" derives from the Greek, meaning "to form" or to "mold," and although synthetic plastics are employed in some of its procedures, use of the word as a medical term precedes its industrial usage by over half a century. The German surgeon Karl Ferdinand von Grafe wrote the treatise Rhinoplastik *in 1918, but coinage of the term "plastic surgery" has been attributed to Eduard Zeis, who published it in the title of his* Handbuch der plastischen Chirurgie *(1838).*

The principles of plastic surgery were developed during thousands of years of trial and improvement. The first record of this knowledge has been traced to the famous Hindu surgeon Susruta, who described the reconstruction of noses using flaps of tissue from the adjacent cheeks; in Susruta's India (perhaps as early as 600 BC) the removal of a portion of the nose was a common punishment for female adultery. From China in the 3rd century BC emerged descriptions of surgery for the correction of such birth defects as split lips. Ceisus in the 1st century AD and Gaten in the following century described facial rebuilding techniques and are credited with the introduction of plastic surgery to Europe. Gaspere Tagliacozzi of Bologna, author of the first textbook of plastic surgery in 1597, gained fame for his rebuilding of noses using arm tissue. This was not an uncommon need at that time because the nasal tip was frequently damaged in sword fights.

Research in plastic surgery began in Italy in 1804 when Giuseppe Baronio experimented with grafts of skin, using sheep as an experimental model. Many 19th-century European and American surgeons published articles on topics that were to become the nucleus of the specialty, such as facial reconstruction, palate repairs, lip closure, and burn treatments. John Jones, the first professor of surgery at King's College (now Columbia University), New York City, introduced the techniques of plastic surgery to the American colonies with the publishing of his Plain Concise Practical Remarks, on the Treatment of Wounds and Fractures (*1775*).

Much experience was gained from the treatment of casualties of the U.S. Civil War, during which was recorded the performance of 32 plastic operations. Contributions to Reparative Surgery (*1876*), *written by New York surgeon Gurdon Buck, was based largely on his experiences as a consultant to the Union Army. John Roe of Rochester, N.Y., introduced aesthetic surgery to the U.S. in 1887, when he described a method of rhinoplasty, or plastic surgery of the nose, using internal incisions. The first full-time plastic surgeon, John Staige Davis of Baltimore, published* Plastic Surgery *in 1919, and a veritable explosion of information and advances followed the founding of the American Association of Plastic Surgeons two years later, the first such society in the world.* Plastic and Reconstructive Surgery, *the first journal devoted exclusively to the field, began publication in 1946.**

Terminology . . .

By now you are familiar with most of the technical terminology in cosmetic surgery, which includes essentially six operations: face, eyes, nose, ears, breasts, body (tummy and thigh).

If you need them for reference, here they are:

Nose: (rhinoplasty)

Eyelids: (blepharoplasty)

Facelift: (rhytidoplasty)

Ear: (otoplasty) This is most often done to realign protruding ears.

Breast: There are three kinds of cosmetic breast surgery: breast reduction, breast augmentation, breast-lift.

* Peter McKinney, *"Plastic Surgery,"* 1973 *Yearbook of Science and the Future,* Encyclopaedia Britannica.

Body: (lipectomy) Removal of abdominal fat. This is an umbrella term for the correction of a grossly sagging stomach, the so-called "apron stomach," and of severely drooping buttocks.

Costs . . .

Fees for cosmetic surgery are usually higher in New York and Los Angeles. You can count on an average of $5,000 or $6,000—and up, depending on how much you have done. An eyelid or nose job will cost an extra $1,000 to $3,000. In addition, there will be an anesthesia fee (usually from $300 to $600) and a fee for the use of the office operating-room facilities (usually from $300 to $500) if you choose to have the operation in the doctor's office rather than the hospital. And hospital costs are even higher. In addition there's the minimum $100- to $200-a-day post-operative care in your recuperative hideaway hotel, motel, condo, or villa.

Prices are somewhat lower in cities like Atlanta, Houston, and St. Louis. But nowhere can you get a *good* facelift at bargain-basement prices. So forget that.

Also, of course, you can't put your facelift on your Visa or Master Charge credit card—nor even on a routine credit-billing basis as you do with other doctors.

For cosmetic surgery it's cash in advance and you sign a written consent waiver which releases the doctor in case you have an inclination to sue. Many do.

Medical insurance does not cover facelifts but according to a new wrinkle in the IRS, they're now a legitimate deductible medical expense. I wouldn't bank on it.

24

How Do I Find the Right Doctor?

This of course is the crucial question. It's what this book is all about.

ARE YOU *SURE* YOU WANT THAT LIFT?

Many are already sure. Either they do or they don't, for whatever reasons.

Many also are so sure and so eager that they'll take the first doctor handy.

But for those of us still weighing the pros and cons, the answer hinges on finding the right doctor. At least for me it does. And it should for you.

The guidelines I'm going to give you will be X-rated by the AMA and ASPRS, whose official advice pamphlets on the subject specialize in doctors' double-talk and the big run-around.

I'll preface my Q & A here by bringing you up to date on an interesting development that has happened to me during the preparation of this book.

Dozens of people have asked my opinion on what I think of facelifts in general, meaning do I approve or disapprove of it (facelifting). As a writer it isn't my prerogative or responsibility to tell readers whether they should or shouldn't have a facelift. It is very much a matter of personal and individual decision, and one person has as much right *not* to want it as the next one has to want it.

My purpose is to try to help you decide whether you're *sure* you want it, if you're in limbo between yes and no. My responsibility is to present the facts—all sides—as accurately, conscientiously, and objectively as possible. But in investigating the facts I have reached certain conclusions of my own which are frankly not at all objective because they pertain to me personally—whether *I'm* sure *I* want a facelift.

And I can tell you one thing for sure: I am far *less* sure now in these final chapters than I was in the beginning.

This has nothing whatsoever to do with the facelift operation itself and certainly nothing to do with any moral judgment in the matter. I don't think it's wrong or sinful to have a facelift; I don't think it's sheer vanity to want to look better, to improve your appearance with a facelift. The truth is, I'm even more sold on it now than I was when I started researching the subject.

But I'm *less* sold on the doctors who do it.

The truth is, I had already made up my own mind that I was going to have a facelift. Now I'm not so sure.

I've decided to keep my wrinkles until I find the right doctor, and with the luck I've had so far that might be a couple of reincarnations from now.

Don't let all of this discourage *you*. There are many competent, qualified, good doctors around. Trying to find the right one for *you*, or for me, is the problem.

Even though the facelift business is monopolized by interlopers and charming con artists, many people are willing to check out a doctor's background. Following are some of the questions they ask—and answers supplied by doctors I've interviewed, as well as official medical guidelines. (You'll get the NLB guidelines in the next chapter.)

Where is the best place to go for a facelift? Is it necessary to go to a large city—New York, Los Angeles?

There are more cosmetic surgeons in the larger metropolitan areas and in the beauty and fashion centers of the world—New York, Los Angeles, London, Paris, Rome. But you should be able to find a good plastic surgeon in most major cities of a million or more population. You're not apt to find one in small towns. There wouldn't be much demand for a cosmetic surgeon in Broken Bow, Nebraska, for instance.

Are there better doctors abroad? Are their techniques better? How would I be sure if I went to Argentina or Switzerland, for example?

One of the top plastic surgeons in the United States tells me that one of the best men in the world with *noses* is in Lucerne, Switzerland. But his fee is $6,000. How does that grab you? The going rate here is between $2,000 and $3,000, though there is no "standard" price in any area of cosmetic surgery.

Over-all, virtually every doctor I interviewed, including many who were foreign born, with training and practice in Europe before coming here, said that medical training and techniques are far superior in the United States. Every country has its superstars—but people from abroad come here to study. And people from here go there for facelifts. Paris and Tahiti are (as this is written) the two most popular places to go (abroad) because (a) the price is right (or at least better) and (b) the cosmetic surgeons are more aesthetically oriented, as well as skilled, and (c) well—the place is right, too.

Is there any way of having a facelift done if you can't afford the usual prices, yet don't want to settle for what might be less than a good doctor?

Yes. You can have it done in a medical school residency teaching program. Chicago has some of the better residencies in the country for plastic surgery, with five medical schools and excellent hospital training programs and facilities. New

York and Los Angeles medical schools also have residency training programs in cosmetic surgery. This means that the doctor doing his residency in plastic surgery in a certain hospital may be allowed to perform a facelift operation under the supervision of his teacher. Some residents-in-training are very good at facelifts. But the operation is done only as a *teaching* procedure, so don't get your hopes up. It isn't the same as getting your hair permed in a beauty school.

Is a background in art essential to good cosmetic surgery?

Perhaps not essential but it helps. It stands to reason that a doctor whose specialty is reshaping faces should have an interest or background in art and symmetry. And it's amazing the number of plastic surgeons who do have at least an artistic background. "I don't think they can be good cosmetic surgeons unless they have a certain appreciation of art, and the ability to conceptualize, visualize before the surgery," says one.

New York's Dr. Richard Stark, a highly respected plastic surgeon, is also an accomplished painter. Chicago's Dr. Peter McKinney comes from four generations of artists; his mother was Esther Williams, a well-known American painter, his father a museum director and author of four books on American art. . . . Rio's Dr. Ivo Pitanguy is president of the Rio Museum of Modern Art and of the Franco-Brazilian Cultural Institute. . . . Dr. Robert A. Franklyn, one of Hollywood's most famous plastic surgeons, says, "The skill to be a cosmetic surgeon is something you have to be born with. They can train you at Mayo's under fifteen different professors, and they still can't turn out a beautiful face or a good pair of breasts. . . . I discount any specific type of training or schooling. All we ask of our trainees is that they have a great artistic ability. Did Picasso or Rembrandt go to the same school? Does it even matter?"

As for those foreign-born and -trained doctors who claim they're better at cosmetic surgery because their approach is more artistic and American doctors more commercial, it has been my personal observation that the foreign facelifters in the United States catch on to our fast-buck approach pretty fast.

If I do not live near a large metropolitan area, how would I go about finding a plastic surgeon?

Get in touch with the American Society of Plastic and Reconstructive Surgeons, whose headquarters are in Chicago. Most states also have their own ASPRS. The ASPRS has a *referral service* which will give you names of three or four doctors in the areas closest to where you live. If you live in Utah, for instance, they'll give you names of doctors in vicinities nearest your address—but this doesn't mean they're *good* cosmetic surgeons. It only means they've completed their post-medical school training and passed their Board examinations. An ASPRS gold seal of approval does *not* guarantee that any doctor is a whiz kid at facelifts. Neither do other medical referrals. You can check with your county medical society or consult the Directory of Medical Specialists, which lists all Board certified specialists in the United States, and is available in most libraries. Or you can check with your internist (GP), if you have one, who in turn will probably consult the Directory of Medical Specialists or the county medical society and give you the same names the ASPRS gave you.

There's a million-to-one chance you might find an internist who is interested and knowledgeable enough about cosmetic surgery to recommend a good facelifter, though I wouldn't bet money on it.

How will I know if he is qualified or not? Where and how can I check on him?

It's easy enough to check out his medical-academic qualifications through official sources such as those listed above; to check out his expertise at facelifting you'll need sources other than medical referrals (his patients).

Should I avoid doctors who advertise?

Yes. Like scorpions.

Are there consulting fees?

Yes, from an average of $35 to $75 per consultation. And be prepared for a whole bunch of consultations while you're looking for a doctor, and two or three after you find the right one.

Would I dare ask to see degrees or proof of his ability?

By all means, you *should* ask to see all his credentials. Then take them all with a grain of salt. They are not proof of his ability as a cosmetic surgeon.

Is it possible for me to see other patients he has worked on? If so, can I talk to those patients?

Though some patients absolutely refuse to discuss the operation with anyone, every plastic surgeon should be able to provide you with names of patients who are willing to talk about it confidentially—to help you.

However, in making your evaluation, it is important to remember: *Both doctors and patients can stack the deck in their favor.* The doctor can show off only his good results (as is always done with photographs); he's not going to pull the bad ones out of the closet and let you talk to them. Similarly, his "good results," the patients who are ecstatic over their facelifts, usually become evangelists for the doctor who did it. Until the next time. Among the chic chicks who go in for repeats—another lift or tuck-up—the switcheroo in surgeons is like musical chairs. Their doctor endorsements should be weighed carefully.

Would it be ethical to bring my regular doctor in on the case?

This is a peculiar question but since someone asked it, others may wonder too. I have never heard of anyone's "regular" doctor, presumably an internist or GP, being brought in on a facelift case. I doubt if either the GP or facelifter would be enthusiastic about such a liaison, though all sorts of other "regular" doctors such as cardiologists have had to be brought in during emergencies, like a heart attack during a facelift.

Could I question the AMA on the doctor's ability and qualifications, or would they answer?

Save your time. You'll get nothing but the runaround here. However, it might be worth your while to consult the AMA's physician listings roster regarding a doctor's background. Let's say he was trained at State U., interned in the Navy, took his residency at a VA hospital in Oklahoma. Would you want him to do your facelift?

ASPRS Summary: (Not endorsed by NLB.)

Excerpts from pamphlets given out by the ASPRS give these guidelines:

• Don't "finger shop" for a surgeon in the Yellow Pages. Instead, consult your family physician because if you have confidence in him you will have confidence in the surgeon he recommends. (Not always.)

• Consult the Directory of Medical Specialists, etcetera . . . (Not much help.)

• Ask to see the surgeon's credentials, etcetera. ("The doctor will be pleased you are concerned enough to ask." Oh yes?)

• Ask the doctor which hospital he is affiliated with. It is a good indication of competence. (Not necessarily so.)

The ASPRS says it's preferable to use these guidelines rather than to select a surgeon on the recommendation of a friend who has had a similar operation.

Above all—*Don't shop. Ask your family doctor.*

They've got to be kidding.

Yet every popular magazine article and book on the subject follows the ASPRS party line and Hippocratic hype.

Their guidelines are not only not very helpful, but self-serving, deceptive, misleading, and a grave injustice to anyone who is giving thoughtful consideration to having a facelift or any other form of cosmetic surgery.

Anyone but the hopelessly harebrained will indeed want and make an effort to check out a doctor's background and credentials through regular channels. But specialty boards do not guarantee or even promise you a good operation. In the final essence a surgeon's background gives you an indication that he has a certain basic competence, that he isn't a quack, that he is equipped and prepared to take care of you. But when you start to look beyond that, you must look at the results the man gets.

This will entail a great deal of shopping around.

And any time you run across that retreaded anachronism, "Don't shop. Ask your family doctor," my advice is to throw the book away.

In the first place, your family doctor probably isn't interested enough to know a halfway decent facelift when he sees one, much less recommend a cosmetic surgeon.

Most people do have a family physician, a GP or internist, but generally, physician attitudes toward facelifts are such that many people are afraid to ask.

So why do all the medical guidelines tell you to ask your family doctor and don't shop around?

Because organized MDs are a very tight and uptight fraternity; when they're not knifing each other, they can be obsessively protective. They stick together.

According to the ASPRS guidelines, you're not even supposed to shop around among your friends. "A friend's referral is *not* the best," they say.

It may not be the best but it's probably better than a GP's.

The appalling and shameful truth is that the ASPRS continues to perpetrate their don't-shop-ask-your-family-doctor line when they know—or hasn't the news caught up with them?—that their own members most certainly do recommend shopping around, getting advice from others; and that nationwide in major cities *75 to 80 per cent of all cosmetic surgeries are from patient referrals, only 20 to 25 per cent from physician referrals.*

In major population centers such as New York, Chicago,

and Los Angeles it is easier to find an internist who is knowledgeable about cosmetic surgeons and perhaps even willing to recommend one. Certainly he can't go too far wrong in recommending the top one, two, or three plastic surgeons in a city; usually their names are well-known nationally, their reputation and ethics beyond reproach; they are highly respected and esteemed by their peers, and often well connected with major medical centers and teaching hospitals.

I have interviewed many of them for this book. They are all members of the ASPRS. Virtually every single one of them emphasized the importance of what in essence *is* "shopping around" for a doctor.

Chicago's Dr. Peter McKinney says: "You should try to talk to at least two Board certified plastic surgeons."

New York's Dr. Victor I. Rosenberg, director of plastic surgery at Beekman Downtown Hospital, sums up what I found to be the majority opinion, with this advice:

"The best way to find a plastic surgeon is by recommendation from someone you know who has had an operation performed and who is pleased with the results—and you liked the result too."

Failing that, he adds dutifully, you can ask a family doctor for the names of plastic surgeons or write to the ASPRS in Chicago.

I have a more expedient solution which is so simple I'm surprised the ASPRS hasn't thought of it.

But before I come to that, here's an important tip on that first item in the ASPRS guidelines: "Don't 'finger shop' for a surgeon in the Yellow Pages." Again they're off-base. (They must have a closed-shop hang-up.) Any reasonably intelligent person knows that the best way to find the best of any consumer product is by shopping around—*and this includes the very important process of elimination.* The Yellow Pages of your local telephone directory can be a very handy guide to the right doctor by steering you away from the wrong ones. Turn to *Physicians and Surgeons,* examine their specialties, cross-check the names listed under Plastic Surgery with those under Otolaryngology (ear, nose, throat), Orthopedic Surgery, Dermatology, Opthamology, Acupuncture, and so on. Also check the advertisements in this medical section of the Yellow Pages. I highly recommend "finger shopping" in the Yellow Pages as one of your first steps—and a relatively easy one—in the important process of elimination. The last doctors to choose for a facelift are those with the biggest ads and their names in bold type in specialty categories where they don't belong. Cross them off your list. (Review Chapter 13, The Big Hype.)

CROSS EXAMINATION:

If You Ask Me, Straight Talk...

25

Ask Your Hairdresser...

How would *I* go about finding a doctor to do my own face? Well, I'll tell you. I'd ask my hairdresser. And my manicurist. Then I'd switch beauty shops and ask again. And again. I've switched beauty shops dozens of times during the preparation of this book.

So okay, it will be banned by the ASPRS. Terrific. They should all go to the beauty shop more often to see their little malfunctions.

Of all the absolute, utter nonsense put out by the ASPRS propagandists is this typical little gem:

"It [the facelift] is, after all, surgery—a medical and not a beautician's procedure, and any sensible woman will consult her internist and not her hair-dresser, her dressmaker, her women friends" etc. . . .

Succinctly, nuts!

Any sensible woman knows that her hairdresser knows more about facelifts than her GP, and anyone who tries to tell you any differently is daffy.

Obviously the "experts" who try to feed you this drivel do their own shampoos and hair-sets at home.

Otherwise they would know that the beauty shop is a most remarkable emporium for gossipy information-gathering of the most secretive nature; and who has or hasn't had a facelift or needs one or is going to have one, and when and where and by whom has long been the most popular topic of conversation.

The beauty shop is in fact a fountainhead of facelift information—*including the youth doctors' mistakes*.

Your internist won't tell you (even if he knows) but your hairdresser will.

The plastic surgeons won't tell you but the hairdressers will. You expect doctors to admit their mistakes? Certainly not those making a pitch for your face.

Beauticians do not pretend to be facelift doctors, nor to know their medical techniques. Generally they know nothing about a doctor's medical background or so-called "qualifications," and they couldn't care less. They have no medical ax to grind; they're not in the business of recommending doctors.

But they *do* know a facelift when they see one, which is more than some GPs know. They are well qualified by the nature of their beautician's craft to know a good facelift from a bad one; many are experts in being able to tell at a glance whether you've had a facelift or not, even though you may have had it fifteen or twenty years ago, and even though they may never have worked on your hair.

They become quite skilled facelift judges by dint of sheer numbers if nothing else. In many beauty shops, from 50 to 75 per cent of the customers have had facelifts. The percentages are probably higher on the West Coast and certainly higher in Palm Springs.

To say that any "sensible" woman will *not* consult her hairdresser doesn't make any sense at all.

I say that any sensible woman who doesn't already have a hairdresser would be well advised to get one immediately; if you don't like the way he styles your hair, stick it out until you get the *information* you want, which won't take too long unless you're deaf, dumb, and blind. Then switch to another hairdresser and repeat. It will save you time and money in the long run. A hairdresser's fees usually are less than those for a facelift consultation. And meanwhile you may come out of the beauty shop looking better than if you'd been to either a plastic surgeon or GP.

If you're seriously considering a facelift, my number one rule of advice is: *Gather as much information as possible on the doctors you may be considering.*

The best and quickest source of information is the beauty shop. It's also the most intimate and therefore, in my opinion, the most honest information you'll get—not only from the hairdressers and manicurists but from all of those customers sitting next to you, in curlers in front of the mirror, or under the hair dryer.

Anyone who doesn't know that this is where all intimacies, human foibles and yearnings, regrets and hallelujahs, are aired, bared, and shared, is simply living on another planet.

If the medical authorities on facelifts have not heard about the beauty shop as a prime source of information, then I would say they're not Board qualified to know what they're talking about.

As I mentioned earlier, beauticians—hairdressers—are usually the first to see the results of a doctor's work. Many are called to the patients' homes, or to the recovery ranchos, condos, villas, or spas to do their makeup, fix their hair, camouflage the bruises and hide the scars, and make them presentable for their first appearance before family and friends or in public.

Beauty operators also have the advantage of observing the results of a doctor's work over a long period of time—if their customers don't switch hairdressers. They know where the scars are; it's their job to hide the scars with the hair-do. They know if the scars are healing or not healing; they see the infections and complications; and in all too many cases it's the hairdresser who has to hustle his client off secretively to another doctor for repairs.

In general he's better informed than her GP in an emergency.

• How many women have weekly standing appointments with their GPs as compared with their hairdressers?

• How many GPs care about the scars under your eyebrows or behind your ears?

Internists and GPs, let's face it, are more concerned with your blood pressure and bowel movements than your facelift.

My personal guidelines to a good facelift doctor:

1. *Start in your beauty shop.* It's the quickest, closest, most reliable and *unprejudiced* source of information available.

2. Then—*CHECK IT OUT!*

If you prefer to ask your family doctor (if you have one) or internist or a dozen or so plastic surgeons, go ahead, ask them first, then check them all out at the beauty shop, where only they know the secrets that even your best friends and doctors won't tell you.

Many people don't like to admit they've made a mistake with their doctor. Many are still enamored of the doctor in spite of his mistakes. They'll tell you, "Well, he didn't do enough here—or a little too much there—but *he's going to do it over again.*"

I've heard that same old tune until it's pouring out of my ears.

The most helpful role of the beauty shop is that it gives you specific points of reference quicker and faster and more honestly than you'll find anywhere else.

The most important point to remember is: *Don't swallow anything hook, line, and sinker. Check it all out.*

But at least you have starting points for the check-out.

• Keep your eyes and ears open.

• Listen. Ask questions. Not conspicuously; subtle probing is often best.

• Make a mental note of all the name-droppings, Drs. X, Y, and Z, and what those ladies under the hair dryer said about them.

• Then *CHECK THEM OUT*.

You do this with your own personal follow-up investigation which isn't all that difficult when you start in the beauty shop. First of all, most women you meet there will be willing to talk to you privately if they are approached discreetly. Some have no inhibitions about talking to everyone within hearing distance about their facelifts. Others are more reticent. If it's someone you don't know, ask your hairdresser to tell her that you're thinking about having your face done and that you're scared—many women are at first—and would like to talk to someone who has been through it. Also ask your hairdresser *and* manicurist (they often become confidantes of their clients) if they know anyone else who'd be willing to talk to you about their experience. Ask your friends to ask *their* hairdressers.

In no time at all you can have more appointments lined up than you could have from any doctor—and the random sampling will give you a much broader scope of comparison, more information, more differing opinions, and therefore a more objective appraisal than you would have if you talked to only those people the doctor picked out for you.

You'll see not only the good results but the bad ones too —or at least you'll hear about them. Many women are eager and willing to tell you about the doctor's boo-boos, or how many times they had to go back to have something "fixed," or whether they had a repair job by another doctor. They'll tell you whether they had an infection or complication; some blame the doctor, some blame themselves. Usually they'll talk to you frankly if you assure them the information will be kept in confidence—you only want to know for yourself to help you decide whether to have a facelift.

In all of these woman-to-woman talks you'll get a real bonanza of tips, many of which can be very valuable to *you* if you know how to use them.

Be wary of the woman who is overly enthusiastic or overly critical. She might be ecstatic about her doctor because he's the "in" man for facelifts right now; or she might be the Virgo nitpicker type who wouldn't be happy with any doctor.

Anyone who is a halfway decent judge of human nature will know how to examine and analyze and sift all the tidbits of information gleaned from these confidential girl-talk sessions.

Some important questions for you to ask, in case they forget to volunteer the information: *What kind of care did the doctor provide in the first few days or week or so after the operation? Were you left alone or was there a nurse or attendant with you or on call? Did the doctor come to see you? Could he be reached when you needed him?*

It may come as a surprise to three very reputable, prominent, and highly qualified plastic surgeons whom I was seriously considering for my own facelift—after personal investigations and consultations with them—that all three have been eliminated from my list because they were "out of town," or unavailable, when patients developed complications and needed them.

It may also come as a surprise to them that this personal process of elimination started with my eavesdropping in *beauty shops*—and then checking out what I heard.

Sample: A distraught woman staggered through the back door of her beauty shop, called for her hairdresser and manicurist to come into the dressing room, removed her dark glasses and head scarf, and showed them her face. It was a mess. An infection had developed in one of the wounds, she had been trying for two days to locate the doctor, an office assistant had treated the wound, it was worse; she wanted another doctor—fast. None of her friends or family knew she'd had the operation; she didn't know who to ask about another doctor except her hairdresser and manicurist. They found one to take care of her. She recovered.

But the incident left some of us who knew about it in a state of shock and sudden disenchantment with the doctor who had an excellent reputation and up to then was a favorite candidate in my book to do my face.

Sample: (Mentioned earlier in a different context.) A doctor's aide drove a woman to his recovery condo the day after her operation. En route he hit a bump in the road, knocked her out of her seat and the stitches out of the incision under her ear. Same scenario: the doctor was out of town, the wound treated by an aide, infection, etc. When I visited her in her condo the poor woman was practically scared to death, and I would have been too. She was from out of town, was left entirely alone in the condo—except when a nearby health spa director popped in occasionally with a take-home hamburger and chocolate malt.

There are many—in my opinion entirely too many—such samples of doctor neglect and inadequate care and attention to patients after a facelift operation; and I'm not talking here about the doctors who are outright quacks or con operators but those with fine reputations, whose credentials check out, and who also by and large turn out good results with their facelift operations. Their patients' mishaps, injuries, infections, and other complications in the early days of post-operative recovery may not be major from the doctor's point of view but they can be very distressful to the patient at the time.

You will not learn much about these minor details in your doctor consultations, so you should concentrate on getting yourself well armed with as much information as possible in your round of beauty shops. They're your best steering and clearinghouse when you're seriously sleuthing for a doctor to do your facelift.

At the same time, of course, you should be checking out the background and credentials of the doctors whose good results have impressed you the most. You can do this checking through the "regular" channels, i.e., library medical directories, professional associations, or your good old Family Doctor.

Eventually you will narrow your list of favorite candidates for *your* facelift to perhaps three or four, or five or six. I personally recommend no less than three. And then you're ready to embark on your rounds of *doctor consultations*.

I know some women who have come to town (Palm Springs) with scheduled consultation appointments with three doctors, and after the first one, they canceled the other two— they were that sold on *that* doctor.

I know others who after eight or ten or maybe a dozen or so doctor consultations are still searching.

Much depends on the doctor-patient rapport rather than the doctor's technique.

For instance, one of my personal consultations was with a world-renowned plastic surgeon (not in Palm Springs) whose name is a household word among those "in the know"—and one of the most highly respected among his peers.

In such a jealousy-laden profession I was amazed to hear some top-notch plastic surgeons say that if they wanted a facelift themselves, they would go to *him*. It's the ultimate recommendation. (And don't ask me for his name; he's already booked up for years.)

Yet, after my consultation with him, I came out knowing that I wouldn't let him touch my face with a ten-foot pole. He may turn out the world's best facelifts technically—and safely —but his manner is brusque, curt, disdainful, and he is disinterested in facelifts. He's prouder of his cleft palates.

There are many considerations that can tip the balance scale even among the world's finest facelifters. Your rapport with a doctor is among the most important.

During your consultations with the doctors, here are some questions you should ask:

• Where was he trained? Where did he study? What is his experience? These are basics. Even if you've already checked this out, ask the doctor. Pay attention to his answers, his mood and manner when he replies. It may irritate him to be quizzed. He may try to infer that he's Board certified when he's still only a candidate for certification. Some are candidates for years and never Board certified. Some non-Board certified do better facelifts than many of those Board certified. The difference isn't so much in a doctor's facelifts as his honesty. You can get a dozen or so doctors to do your facelift as well as the one who misrepresents his credentials. That one you should check out. Thoroughly.

• Ask him what hospitals he is affiliated with. Remember, this isn't always a fool-proof indicator. Plastic surgeons who are strictly *cosmetic* surgeons are not always welcomed with open arms in big general hospitals whose job is treating the sick. But if something goes wrong during your facelift operation, you would want to be assured that your doctor can get you into a hospital.

• Ask him how many operations he performs in a week. Quantity may be a valid measure of quality in this instance. I wouldn't choose a doctor who performs more than one operation a day.

• Ask him what areas of cosmetic surgery he specializes in —faces, breasts, bellies, thighs, etc. I would choose one who specializes in facelifts. Not one who specializes in children with congenital defects.

• Ask him about his art background. Is he only a technically competent nip-and-tuck craftsman with the scalpel, or a molder of faces with an artist's aesthetic eye for contours, sculpting, and symmetry?

• And finally, though you can't ask him point blank about his personal habits and lifestyle, you can check him out in other ways on questions such as: Family? Problems? Patient liaisons? Socializing? Boozing?

In most circumstances a doctor's personal life isn't *your* business and vice versa unless it affects the end results of his work. If it's your face he's working on, you don't want someone who's tipsy with the scalpel. So, while he's checking on *your* id and ego, keep your antenna tuned to his. And don't trust the guy who greets you in white surgical cap and gown and fresh-from-the-ranch boots. At least he should have them polished.

26

Wrap-up, Your Turn

Now it's Q & A time from the audience. What would *you* ask *me* if you had the chance on a personal one-to-one basis? I can guess some of the questions; they've been asked many times before. Many of the answers you'll find if you read between the lines in certain chapters of this book.

For a summing-up, here are from-the-heart answers to questions that may have left you with lingering doubts:

Would you *personally have a facelift?*

Yes. Definitely. When I find the right doctor. Not before.

Would you have it done in a doctor's office or hospital?

If I had to choose between having it done in a hospital or not at all, I would skip it. (See Chapter 19, "Hello, Room Service? . . .") But in choosing a doctor's private office-clinic setup, I would request to see his operating room and facilities and make certain that they're as good as those in a hospital. (Many are better.) Also I'd make certain the doctor has enough hospital connections—and clout—to get me admitted promptly in an emergency.

Would you personally consult your family doctor or internist before having a facelift?

Yes indeed. I already have. Though generally they're not too helpful or supportive in the should-I-or-shouldn't-I stages, your own "regular" doctor should be informed when you've finally decided for sure to have a facelift. Mine will be the first to know—in case I need him for an emergency. If your GP disapproves to the point of refusing to have any part of it, and some do, get yourself a standby doctor who can take care of you when your facelifter leaves town. *Personally I would not entrust my face to any cosmetic surgeon without notifying my own doctor.*

You may wonder—Why such caution? We don't notify our GPs when we have a gall bladder removed. No, because the GPs—or internists—notify us. They recommend the specialist to do it and that's it. You're not likely to get such authoritative recommendations for wrinkle removing even among your best-friend GPs. So it's a do-it-yourself decision process and when you've made up your mind, *do* by all means *tell* your friendly family physician, or internist, or pediatrician, or any other MD you may be on good terms with, so maybe he'll patch up those little mishaps like stitches knocked out while your facelifter is out of town.

This is not meant to be disparaging, only realistic. If I have my face done, I'll make sure there is another doctor available when the facelifter isn't.

What kind of post-operative recovery places do you recommend?

Recovery ranchos with exotic wildlife like llamas are fun; condos are luxurious and lonely; hotels have room service; health spas can give you a real uplift while you're mending from your facelift. It depends on how much privacy you want for how long, and how much you can afford. I'd choose the health spa or hotel with room service if I could afford it. But I'd still make sure there's a doctor on call if my stitches come out.

Where would you go for your facelift—any special city or country?

Since I live in California and loathe flying, I'd prefer to have it done here. But my hopes for this have been dismally diminished in proportion to the ratio of my research.

Which doctor do you recommend?

None. You do your own investigation and make your own choice.

Which process do you recommend—facial surgery or chemical peel?

Neither. Again, investigate, make your own choice. (See Chapters 8 to 11.) Personally, I am *very* wary of plastic surgeons who do peels along with their surgical lifts, and especially wary of those who try to sell me on a full face peel as an "adjunct" to my facelift; and I certainly would *never* trust my face to a doctor who does a full facelift and full face peel in the same operation. That eliminates another of my favorite candidates who had a fairly good head start on getting my facelift business until I learned about his peels. If I want a peel I'll go to Miami where they know how to do it.

P.S. on Peel . . .

To clarify further my answer on the face peel versus the surgical lift, I do not recommend one procedure over the other but I *do* recommend both equally to anyone who wants a facelift. Both have advantages and disadvantages: the surgical lift doesn't remove deep wrinkles, the deep peel does; with the peel you definitely have to stay out of the sun, which I personally would find difficult, but to many women this doesn't matter.

As for doing the full face peel and full surgical lift in the same operation, this is such a recent, rare—and daring!—innovation that I haven't seen anyone whose lift-and-peel at this point is more than a few months old. All the medical literature warns against it; even plastic surgeons who do small area peels, such as around the mouth and on the forehead to remove frown wrinkles, say that it is extremely dangerous to do the full chemical face peel at the same time as the surgery. My calculated guess is that the doctors now doing the lift-and-peel in the same operation are giving an extremely light peel—to be on the safe side—and that its results won't last long. However, some women may prefer a light peel every year to a deep one that lasts ten years or more. Catherine the Great, empress and tsarina of Russia, was said to have had a peel every year, presumably to stay young and beautiful for all her lovers.

Would you prefer to go to a European or an American doctor for your facelift?

I would prefer a European doctor if I could find one who hasn't caught up with the American modus operandi in the wrinkle racket. I feel that Europeans generally are more knowledgeable in this field, more artistically and aesthetically oriented to cosmetic surgery, more gentle and sensitive in their appraisal, approach, and appreciation of a woman's facial features. The top American plastic surgeons agree that cosmetic surgery is an art form, or a combination of art and science, and that an appreciation of or background in art is essential for good results in a facelift. As I have pointed out earlier, a good many American doctors *do* have an artistic background, and I'm sure they would be the first to agree with me (at least privately) that too many do *not* have. I don't feel that this is necessarily important for good results in other branches of medicine, but it is in cosmetic surgery. It is widely agreed, even among the Europeans I've talked to, that medical training and techniques in plastic surgery are better in the United States than Europe. But generally speaking, I'd put most American facelift doctors (and remember, they're not all plastic surgeons) in the same category with cookie-cutters. They may know the medical techniques, but they're too clinical, too crass, too commercial, too confounded busy chasing the fast buck to be genuinely interested in your face. It's too bad so many of the European lifters have latched on to the American M.O.

And don't get me wrong—some of my best friends are doctors.

Since you're so down on facelift doctors generally, how do you expect to find one to do your face?

Don't worry, I'll keep looking. And I'll know when I find the right one. He's the one who'll inadvertently make *me* answer the big question I'm asking *you—ARE YOU SURE YOU WANT THAT LIFT?* I'll know when I'm ready to say Yes. And so will you. As a matter of fact, there are a few doctors mentioned in this book who are among my favorite candidates and who would stand an excellent chance of winning my Yes vote if they were closer to Palm Springs. I'm *not* sure I want a facelift if I have to fly in a DC 10 or a 747 or any of those other Mickey Mouse flying machines to get it.

With the booming business in facelifts practically in my own front yard, and all the opportunities I've had to view the remains, the beautiful doll faces and disasters, wouldn't you think I could have found a doctor by now? The last unveiling party I went to, for instance, was truly a gold mine for comparative research in the field. I counted twenty-five facelifts (including eye and nose jobs) representing the good and bad results of eleven different cosmetic surgeons. And these were only the people I knew personally—as well as their doctors.

It was a large party, more than three hundred guests, many of whom I didn't know, so I can't say what the actual lift count might have been but a count of twenty-five isn't too shabby for conversation openers, especially since the guest of honor was Jolie Gabor, just eighteen days out of her lift-and-peel operation, and her hostess was a lovely lady with partial paralysis of her face and arm from a stroke she suffered during a facelift operation a few years ago.

Jolie's new face, of course, was the talk of the party. It was, to put it mildly, rather spectacular. And taking bows all over the place was her doctor, a handsome young Yugoslavian who is new to Palm Springs but is fast replacing all the others in the affections of facelift candidates who are now clamoring for his lift-and-peel operation.

He is Dr. Borko Djordjevic, barely forty, who readily admits the boldness of his operation but defends it on the basis of the "smashing" results he gets—and I must admit that most of the ones I've seen have looked pretty smashing.

I have seen a lot of his work and have talked to him many times. I've checked out his medical credentials and his office clinic; I'm impressed with his serious, intense, almost fanatic approach to his work; with his artistic and sensitive approach to a woman's face; and with his more than average concern for his patients. But I've told him frankly that I have great reservations about his lift-and-peel operation.

Says Dr. Djordjevic, "It is my brand-new thing. Nobody else does it. Someone has to start something new. Most doctors don't like to change. They're too old to be adventurous. It is my boldness and my concern for my patients that made me want to try it. I am never happy with my work. I'm always thinking of how I can do better, how I can make my patients look better. We need more ingenuity and innovation in this profession.

"Of course I've read all the medical literature. I know it's dangerous if you don't know how to do it. But my chemical formula isn't the same that everyone else uses. I've found that I can take care of the wrinkles at the same time that I'm pulling the skin tight with surgery. The skin can take more beating than most doctors think. I'm writing a paper on it to take before my peers [not published yet] and I think in time this operation will become a common procedure. But someone had to start it and the medical profession has to be ready for it.

"I don't think it's for everybody. Not everyone should have the peel. And other doctors shouldn't try it unless they know what they're doing. That's why I don't want to talk too much about it yet."

As this is written, Dr. Djordjevic has only been doing the lift-and-peel operation for about a year. So far he's had no casualties.

What qualifications do you think are essential in the doctor you would choose to do your facelift?

By now you already know most of them. But to sum them up, I'll start first with the facelifters I would eliminate. They include:

• The outright quacks, charlatans, and those involved in flagrant malpractice cases.

• The fringe interlopers such as ENT specialists and other MDs not qualified to do cosmetic surgery.

• Those who do blatant advertising and merchandising of their product to get patients with pie-in-the-sky promises and claims.

• Those who show me their scrapbooks and especially those who use before-and-after photos in the Yellow Pages, newspaper and magazine ads, and promotional brochures.

• Also I would eliminate any doctor who asks me specifically how young I want to look, or how many years I want taken off, or suggests that I bring in a photograph of myself taken at the age I want to look. Some otherwise well-qualified doctors do this.

• And you also must know by now that I have a very special aversion to and would immediately eliminate any doctor who starts probing my id and ego, analyzing my psyche, hustling me at parties; or who wears fresh-in-from-the-ranch boots in his clinic, or who offers to give me a nose just like Betty Ford's.

Now for the essentials I'd want in the ideal candidate to perform my facelift surgery:

• He should have all the basics, of course, as a bona fide, Board certified plastic surgeon (these are a measurement of his minimum competence), PLUS years of experience as a superbly skilled medical-artist specializing in cosmetic-aesthetic surgery.

• I would choose a surgeon who specializes in facelifts

• Who performs only one operation a day

• Who would perform the entire operation himself and not have an assistant working on one side of my face

• Who would take the time and make the effort to establish a warm and sensitive rapport with his patient.

• He should allow plenty of time for consultations, not make me feel rushed, be willing to answer all my questions without condescension or a bored brush-off.

• Naturally, I would select a surgeon who has not only A-1 operating facilities but top-notch recovery accommodations as well and affiliation with a good hospital in case of emergency.

• And above all I'd choose one who would give me an absolute guarantee of a daily visit from *him—not* his assistant or nurse's aide—during the first week after my facial surgery, and thereafter if needed. This is a routine procedure with most doctors. Many make hospital calls on their patients twice a day. A facelift operation may not be considered major surgery but the fee certainly is equivalent, we have to pay it up front. I think it should include a daily look at my face (whether he likes it or not) by the doctor who took my money; and whether I'm in a hospital, an office clinic, a recuperation condo, villa, or at home, when I'm paying a facelifter, or anyone else, for that matter, I expect service until the job is finished.

27

Are You Ready for
a Facelift?

By now you must have done some serious soul-searching of
your own trying to decide whether to take that plunge with the
surgeon's scalpel. Are you ready for it? Do you realize what
you're getting into and its possible consequences, good or bad?
Are you really prepared to entrust your face—think about it,
Your FACE, and you have only one!—to the hands of a cosmetic surgeon or peeler, for better or worse?

Before taking that important step which could change your
life, here are the most important ten questions you should ask
yourself and try to answer with total honesty. You'll probably
need to go back and review certain chapters to help you answer them.

1. *Do you really want a facelift and if so, why?* Think
about it. In fact, think about it a lot. If you should have any of
those "hidden motivations" the plastic surgeons make so much
of, that's your problem, not theirs. But you should *ask yourself*
your reasons for wanting a facelift. If you're trying to save
your marriage or land a television contract, you'll need more

than a facelift. However, it's quite possible that a facelift can help you land or hold a job in our youth-oriented society, which is a perfectly acceptable reason for having it done.

And there's nothing at all wrong with wanting a facelift for the simple reason that you'd like to look better and feel better. The two go together. But the answer must come from within *you*.

2. *Are your expectations realistic?* Don't expect a facelift to help you enter a beauty contest or make you look like Elizabeth Taylor. The surgeon's scalpel is not a magic wand and the doctor doesn't perform miracles—though some come pretty close! They can actually make your face look much younger, if that's really what you want. But who wants to look twenty-five again? To be realistic, you should expect only to look much better, or the best you can—for the age you *are*.

3. *Is there any one feature about your face that bothers you the most? If it's your nose, then do some extra double-checking before you take the plunge.* Carefully review Chapter 22, The Trouble with Noses. Noses can cause problems. Like the dummy who had hers done, then regretted it because a part of her "heritage" and "roots" had been cut away. If there's the remotest chance you'll miss your old nose, then skip the rhinoplasty, because you can't grow it back the way it was.

4. *Even though you're almost certain you want a facelift, can you handle it in your own social milieu?* Maybe you're from a small town, or a rural or suburban community where facelifts and unveiling parties are not part of the lifestyle. You may be caught in the tell-or-not-to-tell dilemma.

Can you cope with catty friends who say, "I can't tell the difference," or relatives who tell you they liked you better the way you looked before, or people who don't even notice? Or do you want them to notice? If they don't react, you should not blame the doctor for doing a bum job; it's probably the sign of a good job. If you want a drastic change in your face, you can expect drastic reactions from those who knew you before. And remember, even small towns have beauty shops.

Your hairdresser *always* knows, and so will all your friends before too long, so you might as well face up to your facelift and be proud of it. You can't hide it. Stop and think again—are you ready for this?

    5. *Have you considered how your new face is going to look with the rest of your body?* This is a very important question for women in their fifties and sixties and up. A facelift can't change those telltale signs of age on your hands and arms; and it might look incongruous with a bulging belly and thighs and a dowager's hump. The best candidate for a facelift is the woman who takes pride in her over-all physical appearance and keeps herself in good shape with a trim youthful figure. Before investing in a facelift, you might better invest in a gym or spa program of exercise and weight reduction. Many plastic surgeons will not operate on people who are overweight, no matter how much you may want a facelift. But you can always find a money-hungry, tenth-rate facelifter to do the job even if you weigh a ton. It's usually the overweight patients who suffer the strokes and heart attacks on the operating table. Think about it.

    6. *Are you willing to make the sacrifices involved in having a facelift?* These are sacrifices not only in time and money but personal pleasures as well. Are you willing to give up smoking and drinking, fattening foods, outdoor sports, sunbathing? Maybe you don't care for any of these things anyway. Fine. Can you afford the inflationary facelift fee and are you prepared to pay in advance? Remember, you can't buy a facelift on the installment plan or with your Master Charge credit card, and your medical insurance won't cover it. You may have to give up your plans for a nice vacation or a new car in order to pay for your facelift. Is it worth it?

    7. *How well informed are you about the facelift operation?* How much do you know—or want to know—about the surgical procedure itself? If you feel you need further information about the technical aspects of cosmetic surgery, you should go to the library and read the medical literature. If you don't understand it, at least you can browse through and look at the pictures to get a general idea of how the flaps are cut off and the skin tightened and tucked up. Most of the women I've talked to aren't the least bit interested in the technical details; all they want is a doctor they can trust enough to let him do anything he needs to do, as long as they wake up looking younger and prettier. There is much more important and vital information that should concern you than the technical details of facelift surgery. It's all in this book. You may need to read it again to be better informed and prepared.

8. *Are you fully aware of the seriousness of the operation and the risks involved?* Though most people tell you only the bright side, there *are* certain risks involved and some facelift flops. Make sure you've done your homework well by reviewing certain chapters in this book, especially Chapters 12 to 20.

9. *Are you afraid of the operation?* Most people are, so you needn't be ashamed of your fear. I was in the beginning, but not so much now that I know more about it. The important thing is to find a doctor who will help you overcome the fear. And now we come again to that most important, most vital question of all, which you need to answer within yourself—

10. *Have you chosen the right doctor?* I believe you'll find every conceivable kind of guideline to help you throughout this book—from the gobbledygook of organized medicine to the straight talk of individual doctors, patients, and informed lay persons such as beauticians, hairdressers—and, yes, investigative journalists.

Only after you've done your soul-searching, carefully considered and resolved all of the above questions and answers within your own heart, will you be ready to turn over your own face to a doctor for remodeling and rejuvenation.

And you will know, as I will, when you've found the right one. It's when the little voice inside you asks, Am I *Sure?* And the little bell in your head chimes, *Yes.*

Index